COMMON SEXUAL PROBLEMS

...SOLUTIONS

COMMON SEXUAL PROBLEMS
...SOLUTIONS
QUERIES OF OVER 22,000 PEOPLE ANSWERED

PRAKASH KOTHARI MBBS, PhD

UBSPD
UBS Publishers' Distributors Ltd.
New Delhi • Bombay • Bangalore • Madras
Calcutta • Patna • Kanpur • London

UBS Publishers' Distributors Ltd.
5 Ansari Road, New Delhi-110 002
Bombay Bangalore Madras
Calcutta Patna Kanpur London

1st Edition   1987
2nd Edition   1992
First Reprint   1992
2nd Reprint   1993
3rd Reprint   1993
4th Reprint   1994

© *Dr. Prakash Kothari*

All rights reserved. No part of this publication may be reproduced or transmitted in any form or by any means, electronically or mechanically, including photocopying, recording or any information storage or retrieval system, without prior permission in writing from the publisher or in accordance with the provisions of the Copyright Act 1956 (as amended). Any person who does any unauthorized act in relation to this publication may be liable to criminal prosecution and civil claims for damages.

Cover Design : Surendra Sirsat, Rekha Studios, Bombay

Printed at : Tara Art Printers, A-47, Sector V, Noida (U.P.)

The book is dedicated to **KAMDEV**
— The God of Love

The book is dedicated to KAMDE
The Egg of Love

Contents

	Preface to First Edition	ix
	Preface to Second Edition	xi
1.	Sex Education	1
2.	Sexual Myths	9
3.	Male Sexuality	23
4.	Female Sexuality	41
5.	Orgasm	53
6.	Interplay	63
7.	Alternative Orientations	75
8.	Old Age	81
9.	Ill health	87
10.	Marriage	99
11.	Family Planning	105
12.	Aphrodisiacs	119
13.	AIDS	127
14.	Towards Healthy Sexuality	133
15.	Miscellanea	143
	Afterface	155
	Index	157

Preface to First Edition

Since I began writing in popular magazines read by several millions of people from all walks of life, I have come face to face with the problems that people have with the most intimate and important aspect of their life — sex.

I have gone through about ten thousand letters which patients and readers have written to me and which describe symptoms which are remarkably common. "Where, and to whom should we go to discuss problems of sex?" "Is there any one who can really help us?" This is the prevalent plaintive cry in almost all the letters.

Sexuality is a large component of one's personality and does not consist of just the penis and the vagina. In this book, I have attempted to examine various modes of sexual behaviour with a view to clear myths and misconceptions, provide accurate information and thereby help people to develop patterns of sexual behaviour that are healthy, promote happiness and assist them to perform on a higher plane of well-being.

Much has been omitted in this book that could have been included and, it is fervently hoped that nothing has been included which ought to have been omitted.

September 1987
Bombay

Prakash Kothari

Preface to Second Edition

Sex is considered taboo in our orthodox society which prudishly discourages questions about this intimate and integral part of our lives. Hence, one's natural curiosity remains largely unsatisfied and the existing myths, misconceptions and ignorance continue to be perpetuated and passed on from generation to generation, like an inherited social disease.

The prudery and ignorance of this universally practised art defy rationality. Traditionally, sex has never been considered taboo in our society. In fact, the subject has been textually immortalized by ancient Indian geniuses and scholars in masterpieces like the Charak samhita, Shushrut samhita, Kamasutra etc. Thus, it is apparent that knowledge of this subject has been in existence since times immemorial, to quote a french saying, "Rien de nouveau sous le soleil" – nothing is new under the sun. To promote a healthy sexuality this knowledge must reach the masses, a goal, which, though ambitious, is achievable, through sex education.

I have tried to shed light on different aspects of the subject that I believe are important, and have also included some common sexual problems and questions that I have come across in the course of my professional career. Sexual medicine rightfully deserves its long overdue respect and re-cognition as an independent science.

I hope that this bibliographic compilation of my clinical

acumen and knowledge in this speciality succeeds in promoting sexual literacy.

March 1992　　　　　　　　　　*Prakash Kothari*
Bombay

The author is grateful to
Dr. Sujal S. Shah
for editing the manuscript.

1

SEX EDUCATION

Q. What is sex education?

A. Sex education ideally involves education about the anatomy and physiology of the human reproductive system, conception, contraception, psychosexuality, sexual differences and the constituents of love as they relate to sexual behaviour, and is not merely a discussion on how babies are made. It provides a background in which an individual develops into a healthy, responsible adult capable of using the innate sex instinct to the fullest potential, without being obsessed by it. It enables one to recognize and be comfortable with one's sexuality.

Q. Why is formal sex education necessary today ?

A. Recently, due to the principally career oriented approach for economic independence the average age of marriage is delayed. Also with improvement in nutrition and health care, the average age of onset of puberty is earlier and the average life span is extended. Thus, the average potential sexual career of an individual is extended.

The social environment today, though orthodox and prudish, provides constant sexual stimulation. This conflict between sexual drives and social norms generates a tremendous amount of anxiety and sexual frustration which may find expression as increased promiscuity, casual sexual relationships, unwanted teenage pregnancies and an alarming increase in the incidence of sex crimes and sexually transmitted diseases. Rampant myths and misconceptions about sex further complicate the situation. This social problem can only be resolved through comprehensive sex education, which can increase social awareness and improve the social environment. Sex education should be formally incorporated into health education programmes.

Q. What is the right time to start sex education ?

A. There is no right or wrong time to start sex education. It can be started any time after the mind is receptive to conceptual inputs. Even, as the child develops education appropriate to his age may be imparted. Without conscious volition parents are providing sex education to the child from the moment he/she is born. The way the parents hold and touch the child during infancy and the way they both interact with the child and with each other lays the foundation for his future sexual learning. Making the child feel loved and lovable has a profound influence in shaping future attitudes towards sex and sexuality. The way in which the parents relate to each other, their interactions and the day to day life in the family will influence the individual's sense of self-esteem, body image, gender role, family roles as well as the capacity for love, intimacy and sharing.

Q. How should one go about giving sex education ?

A. All children are normally curious about everything including sex. If a youngster does not ask sex-related questions, it is because he/she is given to feel that his/her parents would be uncomfortable in the face of these questions and either would not answer or would not tell the truth. If the parents are comfortable about sex, it should be relatively easy to find an appropriate opportunity to let the youngster know that this is not a forbidden area. For instance, if someone is pregnant; if a female dog has pups; if there is evidence of night emission (wet dreams) the parents could assure the child that its curiosity about these is quite normal. Sometimes a newspaper with an illustrated article on how babies are made or a birth control advertisement, could become a potential source for discussion. Parents should strive to achieve a good rapport with their children and promote a healthy and comfortable parent-child relationship, thus becoming "Approachable Parents."

Q. What is most important for parents to remember while giving sex education ?

A. It is important to encourage the child's question as a constructive curiosity and answer truthfully at a level appropriate to his age. It may happen that when a child asks a question, the parents might not know the answer or, because of their own values, they are unable to reply. At such moments, one may admit "That's a very good question but even I do not know the answer... well, let's find out." Such parents have a better chance of bringing up their children to respect them than those who are not responsive to their children's sexual needs and curiosity; in other words, those who are not approachable. There are some children who never seem to ask questions. It would be an error to assume that since no questions are asked, no answers need to be given.

Q. "Where did I come from?" What is the answer to this question ?

A. When a child asks this question 'Where did I come from?' one can begin by saying "You came from a place, inside mummy's body." If the child can trust you not to be too rigid or hostile in your response to his questions, he will look upon you as a source of wisdom and guidance. Additional information relevant to the question asked may be given as he/she grows and is ready for knowledge suited to that period of development.

Q. Is it harmful if the parent's answers are a little more than what a child can understand?

A. Parents worry a great deal as to whether this knowledge will harm the child. Though we live in a conservative society, scientific knowledge appropriate to the age of the child will not harm the child while ignorance may.

It is better to give the child the basic information asked for in a simple, factual and loving manner. Even if the parent occasionally replies a little more than what the child can understand, there is no harm because this will help in leaving the door open for further questions.

Q. Does giving sex education stimulate urges and sexual desires leading to increase in unwanted pregnancies and venereal diseases?

A. No. Sex education does not stimulate urges and sexual desire. In fact it satisfies one's curiosity with appropriate and correct information enabling one to recognise one's sexuality and sexual orientation.

As mentioned by Milton I. Levine at Cornell University Medical College in New York "There is no evidence whatsoever that sex education is harmful, that it excites curiosity or stimulates sex urges and desires. On the contrary, there is ample evidence that it does help in gaining a wholesome attitude towards sex and understanding of the normal sex attitudes, roles and relationships". He further states that " it may aid our boys and girls to learn to direct their sex impulses with more knowledge and intelligence, to make a correct choice between operating codes of heterosexuality and homosexuality and to recognise and understand those men and women with sex desires and urges which are deviant". In fact, it has been observed that in countries where proper sex education is given, the number of cases of unwanted pregnancies and venereal diseases have reduced considerably.

Q. What should one tell children about sexual abuse ?

A. One should approach the subject directly and objectively giving appropriate and honest information without communicating unnecessary anxiety. This will make the child aware of sexual abuse and enable him to recognise sexual abuse and potential sexual abusers, when he encounters them. School children may be warned not to accept favours from strangers.

In adolescent years, a more frank discussion can take place. A trusting parent-child relationship encourages children to report unusual incidents with other persons, to their parents. In fact, public recognition in the area of child molestation is absolutely essential. Specific incidents which have already occurred should be reported and discussed in a newspapers and on television. This will help in proper handling of sexual molesters.

Q. Can the incidence of sex crimes be reduced by sex education ?

A. Yes. Occasionally when sexual desire becomes intense, and a partner is not available, the only release left is masturbation. Rampant myths about masturbation (that it leads to impotence, homosexuality, tuberculosis etc.) often discourage individuals from indulging in it. In such circumstances, the intensity of sexual desire outweighs moral bindings and one may resort to sexual activity by force i.e. rape. This leads to an increase in sexual crimes. Rapes are also committed due to a common prevalent myth; that a man would be cured of venereal diseases if he has sexual intercourse with a virgin. Sex education, by eradicating these misconceptions, can orient an individual to direct his sexual impulses in a socially acceptable manner.

Q. Can television be helpful in promoting sex education ?

A. Television can be a very effective medium for a multitude of reasons (As it is basically an audio-visual medium it can reach out to the illiterate as well as the literate masses). 'Sex' is considered a taboo in our orthodox society. If sex education were to be given via a public mass medium such as television, it would reflect the government's healthy attitude towards the issue and can decrease the social taboos significantly. Because of its tremendous reach, it will increase public awareness and pave the way towards an honest social environment and sexual literacy.

It is a medium through which education may be passively imparted to the masses, in the privacy of their homes. Thus, shy individuals who are unable to ask questions or seek help, are also provided with the information they desire. Proper information about contraception and sexually transmitted diseases can help in spreading information about Family Planning and also decrease the incidence of STD's. The potential for television, as an effective medium for sex education, is unlimited.

SEXUAL MYTHS

Q. What are the most common sexual myths you come across ?

A. Sexual myths and misconceptions leading to anxiety are the most common sexual problem. Commonest myths are those related to masturbation or dissipation of semen. Other prevalent myths are about celibacy, virginity, passing '*dhat*' or '*veerya*' in the urine, aphrodisiacs etc. These myths are being handed down from one generation to the next and, as a result, many people imagine more problems than they actually have.

Q. What is masturbation ?

A. Masturbation is a deliberate stimulation of the genitals for pleasure, which may or may not be pursued to the point of orgasm.

Q. How do men masturbate ?

A. For men, the commonest method is to fold the palm and fingers over the penis, so as to encircle it and produce friction by to and fro movements, often till orgasm and ejaculation are reached. Variations such as making coital movements against bed clothes, a pillow, pressing against some objects etc. are also reported.

Q. Do women masturbate ? How ?

A. Yes, women do indulge in masturbation. The usual method is by rubbing a finger on the clitoris. The female anatomy permits considerable variations such as thigh rubbing, rubbing clothing between the thighs and making vulval movements, instrumental masturbation by inserting an object into the vagina, striking the clitoris with a water jet etc.

Q. Is masturbation harmful ?

A. Is coitus harmful ? Then how can masturbation be harmful, because essentially masturbation mimics coitus. What the penis does in the vagina during intercourse is the same as what the penis in the hand or the finger does in the vagina during masturbation. It is a myth that masturbation causes acne, insanity, impotence, dark circles around the eyes etc. In fact, it trains the individual's neurological system to respond. It also provides a pleasurable safety valve or outlet for the release of sexual tension, thus reducing the incidence of sexual crimes, unwanted pregnancies and sexually transmitted diseases including AIDS.

Q. Is excessive masturbation harmful ?

A. Firstly, there is no such thing as excessive masturbation. Besides, just as excess of coitus cannot lead to weakness so also an excess of masturbation cannot lead to weakness. The individual mechanics of masturbation and coitus are the same. In masturbation they occur singly and in coitus they occur conjugally. Further, physiologically, it is dis-use which is abuse as it is dis-use and not use which leads to atrophy. Does the tongue become weak in a talkative person and strong if one observes silence ?

I have come across a person who used to masturbate three times a day, regularly for 12 years. When he was examined later, his general condition was good, his blood examination (metabolic profile), and hormonal assays did not reveal any abnormality. His semen analysis was normal, there were no signs suggestive of any disturbance in the genital function and his performance was good.

Q. Is there any treatment for masturbation ?

A. Masturbation per se is not an illness and hence does not require any treatment whatsoever. It requires treatment, if and only if, it becomes obsessive or compulsive and the individual perceives it to be a problem, and not otherwise. In this case the basic problem is psychological and it is the underlying disorder which merits therapy and not masturbation.

Q. How should parents react to their child's masturbation ?

A. Parents are usually disturbed when they find out that their child indulges in masturbation. They should understand that this is a normal stage of psycho-sexual development and a normal expression of childhood sexuality for males and females. It is neither indicative of psychopathology nor of potentially preferential homosexuality in adulthood. They should be very careful not to arouse any fear in the child by scolding or punishing him or making a big issue out of it. In particular the child should not be told any anxiety provoking statements such as, masturbation will damage his sex life or make him insane or lead to genital dysfunction or deformity. Parents should realize that as the child develops it will continue to have strong sexual urges, he/she will be more expressive about his/her sexuality, and will need to find some manner of release. Parents should realize that any anxiety provoking statements at this crucial incipient developmental stage will be detrimental to the child's psyche. They should provide their constructive support if and when the child solicits it, doing no more; otherwise antagonism and failure are likely. The wisdom of this should be apparent to anyone who reflects upon his personal childhood memories.

Q. Does masturbation lead to curvature of the penis ?

A. No. Just as intercourse does not lead to any curvature of the penis, so also masturbation does not lead to any curvature.

Q. Is semen vital ? Does dissipation of semen devitalize a man and promote ageing ?

A. Semen is being secreted day in and day out by the genital apparatus. Sperms constitute less than one percent of seminal fluid, the rest of the fluid is the secretion of the accessory sexual glands, prostate & seminal vesicles. It is being formed for being excreted and cannot be stored even if one wants to do so. Barring conception, semen is not vital. That one drop of semen is equal to hundred drops of blood, which in turn requires a lot of nourishing food, is one of the most rampant sexual myths prevalent.

Q. Does conservation of semen lead to longevity and athletic excellence ?

A. If this had been based on physiological facts, then all bachelors would have become athletes and lived longer!

Q. Does reduced consistency of semen indicate sexual inadequacy ?

A. No. Consistency of semen may vary as it depends upon several factors like period of abstinence, intensity of stimulation etc. However, as a man grows older, consistency does thin out, but it has nothing to do with the individual's sexuality.

Q. Do reduced quantity and change in colour of semen indicate a waning virility ?

A. No. As mentioned earlier, the quantity of semen often depends upon the intensity of stimulation, period of abstinence and age. As a man grows older, the colour of the semen changes from white to light yellow and the quantity may decrease, but the colour and quantity have nothing to do with the sexuality of an individual. Neither does it have any relation to partner satisfaction.

Q. What is 'dhat syndrome' ?

A. Sometime one passes whitish fluid in the urine or while straining at stools. The belief that this fluid is semen is called as the 'dhat syndrome'. This is not a disease and it would not be inappropriate to say that "it exists only in the mind of the beholder."

The physiological sphincter at the neck of the urinary bladder always remains closed and opens only when one is passing urine. Thus, it ensures that normally, urine and semen can never mix together i.e. normally, one cannot pass semen in urine. Sometimes, a physiological alteration in the urinary solutes may change the appearance of urine, making it whitish which is mistaken to be semen by misinformed individuals.

In reality, it is a secretion of the prostate and the urethral glands. When a person squats in the toilet

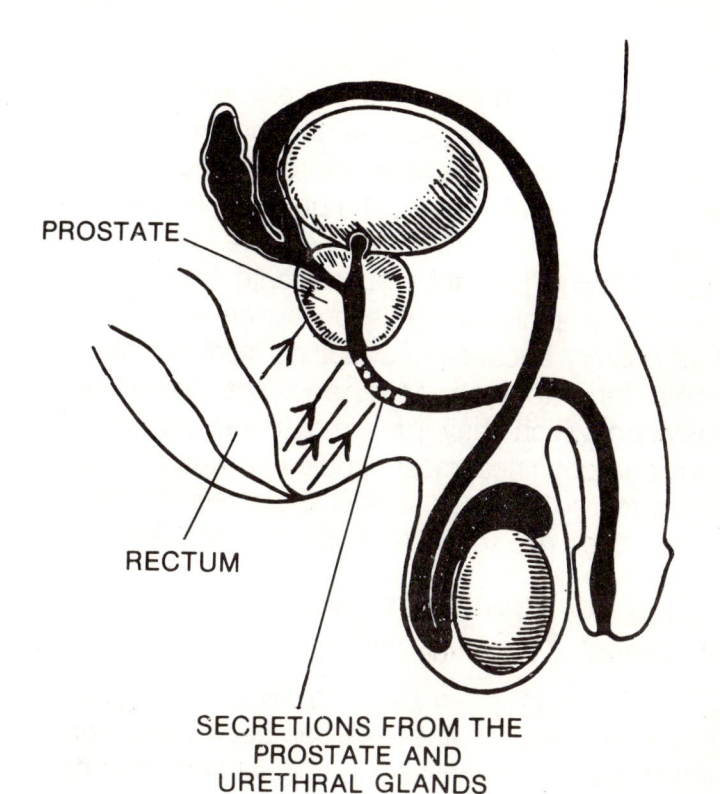

PROSTATE

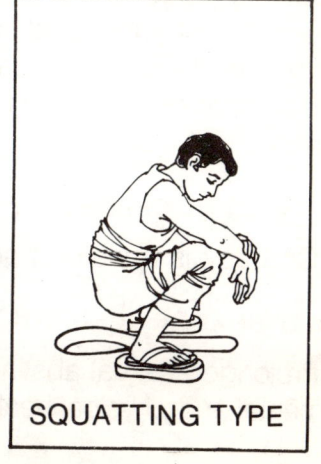

RECTUM

SECRETIONS FROM THE
PROSTATE AND
URETHRAL GLANDS

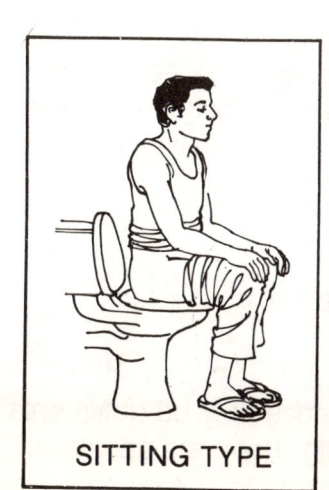

SITTING TYPE

SQUATTING TYPE

and exerts a little pressure, this pressure is relayed from the rectum to the prostate and the urethra, and a few drops of a sticky white secretion accumulate, coalesce and trickle down. The phenomenon is akin to there being 10 drops of perspiration on the forehead being joined by an eleventh and tricking down. In my opinion, this misconception is prevalent in our country because of squatting toilet habits, as people tend to look down and see the sticky substance which they presume to be semen. In developed countries, most people use western style commodes, so they look straight ahead. Hence, 'what the eye does not see, the mind does not know!'

Q. Why do men feel weak after 'sleep emissions' ?

A. Post-emission weakness is totally psychological. Right from childhood the idea has been drilled into our minds that the genitals are special and anything coming out of it is equally special. This misconception about the value of semen, generates tremendous anxiety in an individual leading to neurasthenic symptoms. In fact, the calories lost during sleep emission are equivalent to those contained in a glass of lime juice!

Q. What is celibacy ?

A. Celibacy is a state of sexual abstinence.

Q. Is sexual abstinence advantageous ?

A. Prolonged sexual abstinence may be detrimental to mental and physical health. There are people who are under the impression that sexual abstinence is conducive to human health and happiness. Because of this misguided belief, they make an attempt to conserve the so-called 'energy' by sexual abstinence. The moment they are unable to do this, they get a feeling of guilt and anxiety that they have done something detrimental to their health. When this is repeated several times, the roots of the problem get deeper and deeper. Consistent suppression of the sex drive leads to emotional instability and evokes an abundance of sexual imagery. This usually leads to inability to concentrate, insomnia, irritability and extreme nervousness. The extent of disturbance depends upon the individual's own mental state and the environment. At times, the consistent suppression and continued inactivity of the sex organs lead to diminished ability to function. Besides, it would be a serious mistake to harbour any misconceptions about celibacy as, 'celibacy is not hereditary'.

Q. Is there any relation between the size of the body and the size of the sex organs ?

A. No.

Q. What is the normal length of the erect penis ?

A. Concern about penile size is as old as the human race. The width, length and erection of the penis varies from male to male, as does the length of the nose, the depth and spacing of the eyes and the width of the forehead. The average sexual length of

CLITORIS
URETHRA
VAGINA
ANUS

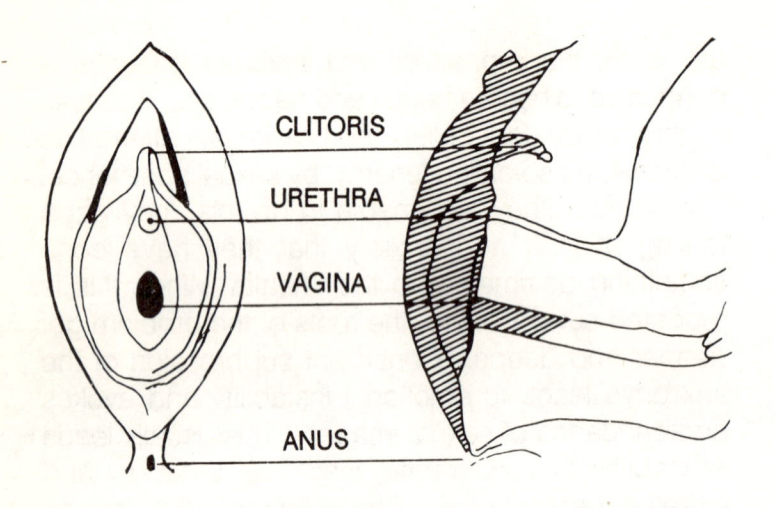

MAXIMUM SENSATION

the vagina is about 15 cms and only the outer third (5 cms) has the maximum nerve endings. The inner two-thirds (10 cms) being virtually insensitive.

If one wants to arouse his partner, he should concentrate on the area where there are maximum nerve endings i.e. the outer lips (labia majora) and the outer third i.e. outer 5 cms of the vagina. Therefore, for female sexual gratification, the size of the erect penis could be anything from 5 cms plus. However, the size of the penis may be an important factor for women who harbour the myth "a man with a large penis can satisfy his partner better than one with a smaller one". Penile size is unimportant for partner satisfaction. "An archer is known by his aim and not by his arrows".

Q. Is the length of the penis in the flaccid state important ?

A. The length in the flaccid state is immaterial... as it is used for urination only. It is the erect penis that is used for performing the sex act and not the flaccid one !

Q. Is the width of the penis important ?

A. No. The vagina is highly elastic. It can expand from the size of the little finger to that of the baby's head. The vagina distends according to the width and size of the inserted penis.

Q. Can a small penis lead to conceptive inadequacy ?

A. No.

Q. Is it advisable to use the vacuum apparatus for enlarging the penis ?

A. No. The use of a vacuum apparatus may prove dangerous and may even lead to fibrous degeneration of the penis.

Q. Is the penis usually inclined towards the left ?

A. Yes, it is true for the majority of men. This is so perhaps because the left testis is lower than the right. Therefore, while wearing their under garments most men adjust their penis on the left side as enough space exists on the left side as compared to the right.

Q. Does a slight curvature of the penis lead to any difficulty in penetration ?

A. No. A slight curvature of the penis either to the left or to the right, is common and does not affect penetration at all. It is a myth that an erect penis should always be at a right angle.

Q. Is it a fact that a women must bleed at the first attempt at sexual intercourse ?

A. No. This usually occurs due to the rupture of the hymen in virgins. However, the hymen may be absent from birth or might rupture while playing games, doing exercises or using tampoons. Hence, a woman need not necessarily bleed at the first attempt at sexual intercourse to prove her virginity. I have seen plenty of marriages going on the rocks because of this misconception.

Q. Do men have a greater sex drive or women ?

A. Sexual urge depends on the individual's sexuality and a greater sex drive is not the prerogative of either sex!

Q. For conception and ideal sexual pleasure, is simultaneous climax necessary ?

A. No. Simultaneous climax in no way ensures conception. In fact the idea of conception often decreases the intensity of pleasure. As for pleasure, it is the pleasure itself that is important. Whether one gets it before, with or after the partner is immaterial.

Q. What is the most dangerous sexual myth ?

A. "A sexologist is always a highly qualified professional".

MALE SEXUALITY

Q. Is it normal for a man to get an erection only after local stimulation?

A. Yes. In adolescence one gets an erection just by sight or erotic thoughts, but after a few years this ability gets reduced and one requires local stimulation to get an erection. This is normal.

Q. Are people with a single testicle impotent?

A. No, one normal testicle secretes enough hormone to maintain an individual's virility.

Q. Does pouring cold water on the testes increase virility ?

A. No. It does not affect the virility of an individual. However, it is believed that an individual with low sperm count and reduced motility of sperms may benefit from this.

Q. What is the most common cause of erectile dysfunctions ?

A. An occasional episode of an erectile failure, due to functional or situational causes like fatigue, tension or pressure to respond and perform, is a very common cause of erectile dysfunctions. This anxiety, if relived during subsequent similar encounters, would result in repeated failures.

Q What is the single best test for differentiating psychological impotence from organic impotence ?

A. If a man can get an erection of adequate quality for a sufficient length of time in any one situation, then the problem is largely psychological and not organic.

Q. Can alcohol lead to impotence ?

A. Yes, as mentioned elsewhere, alcohol can lead to impotence.

Q. How does one treat such impotence ?

A. The treatment programme needs to be tailored to individual needs and circumstances. The physician must determine whether the sexual dysfunction is connected with an isolated episode of drinking or is related to long term intake of alcohol. He must further confirm the normalcy or otherwise of the erectile and ejaculatory components after history-taking and careful physical examination. Depending upon the findings, the physician may inform the patient whether treatment can be implemented or not. If yes, then he may reassure the patient that the sexual function may revert to normal if he completely abstains from alcohol. He should then be made aware that his preoccupation with fear of failure can hamper his sexual responses. Necessary sexual techniques with adequate blending of supportive psychotherapy and behaviour modification may prove extremely beneficial. It is advisable to counsel the partner as well. She could be of great help in the treatment programme if she can understand the situation and is prepared to provide the supportive atmosphere.

Q. What are the most common causes of organic impotence ?

A. Diabetes, vascular disorders and radical surgeries.

Q. Is semen analysis necessary for a patient having impotence ?

A. Absolutely not. The absence or deficiency of sperms does not indicate impotence. Sterility and virility are two entirely different things and depend upon different types of cells present in the testes. Absence or deficiency of sperms does not affect one's virility or potency.

Q. Which investigations are helpful in diagnosing impotence ?

A. Along with metabolic, hormonal and routine physical examination, one should also check the tone of the anal sphincter and bulbocavernous muscle. Evaluation of the autonomic nervous system is a must in cases of impotence.

N.P.T. monitoring: Nocturnal Penile Tumescence monitoring can help in determining whether one is getting erections or not. This, however, does not give any idea about the rigidity of the penis.

E.M.G.: Electromyography studies could help diagnose neurological lesions causing impotence and reduction in pleasure and squirting of semen at the time of orgasm.

Papaverine injection: This involves an injection of papaverine directly in the lateral aspect of the penis (intracavernous). If one gets a good erection then the erectile dysfunction is either due to psychogenic or neurogenic factor or a mild vascular insufficiency. Phentolamine and prostaglandins can also be used.

Doppler examination: This is a non-invasive technique which helps in determining the potency of the superficial and deep vessels of the penis. The quality of the sound and its graphic representation is useful in judging the blood flow. On colour Doppler, blood vessels with blood flow are clearly visualised.

Penile blood pressure: Penile systolic blood pressure (by using a doppler probe and special cuff tied round the penis) divided by the systolic blood pressure of the arm, gives the Penile Brachial Index

(PBI). If it is less than 0.8, it is indicative of vascular insufficiency. This would be further investigated by penile arteriography.

Infusion Cavernosometry and Cavernosography: If the Doppler and other tests are normal, infusion studies with normal saline are helpful in diagnosing venous leaks responsible for inadequate erection. Cavernosography with contrast medium helps in detecting the presence of abnormal draining channels responsible for erectile inadequacy.

Q. What is a penile implant ?

A. A penile implant is a mechanical device used in cases of erectile dysfunction. It is implanted into the penis and is not an artificial penis. There are two varieties of penile implants. One is the semi-rigid implant and the other is the inflatable implant (3 part implant). The details are as follows:

	Semi-rigid	Inflatable
Cost	Less	More
Appearance	Always erect	Under your control
Comfort	Less comfortable	More comfortable
Consistency (Hardness)	Fixed	Adjustable
Complications	Less	More
Surgery	Less time and skill required	More time skill required

Q. Do you recommend the use of a rubber band or the tying of a thread around the penis in cases of impotence?

A. No, this is extremely dangerous, as cases of gangrene have been reported due to this practice.

Q. What about orgasm and ejaculation after implant surgery?

A. If one was able to achieve orgasm and ejaculation before the operation, he will continue to do so.

Q. What are the common causes of pain in an erect penis?

A. Phimosis, paraphimosis, local injuries, ulcers, urethral and prostatic inflammations are known to cause pain on erection. At times in Peyronie's disease or fibrous cavernositis, pain on erection may be a common symptom.

Q. At times, just following an erection or prior to ejaculation, a drop or two of a sticky transparent fluid oozes out from the tip of the penis. Is this normal?

A. Yes. In such situations, the fluid which comes out is the secretion of Cowper's or bulbo-urethral glands. When one encounters a sexual situation, there is a secretion (akin to salivation) from the Cowper's or bulbo-urethral glands which comes out. However, at times it may contain spermatozoa.

MALE GENITALIA
(Sagittal Section)

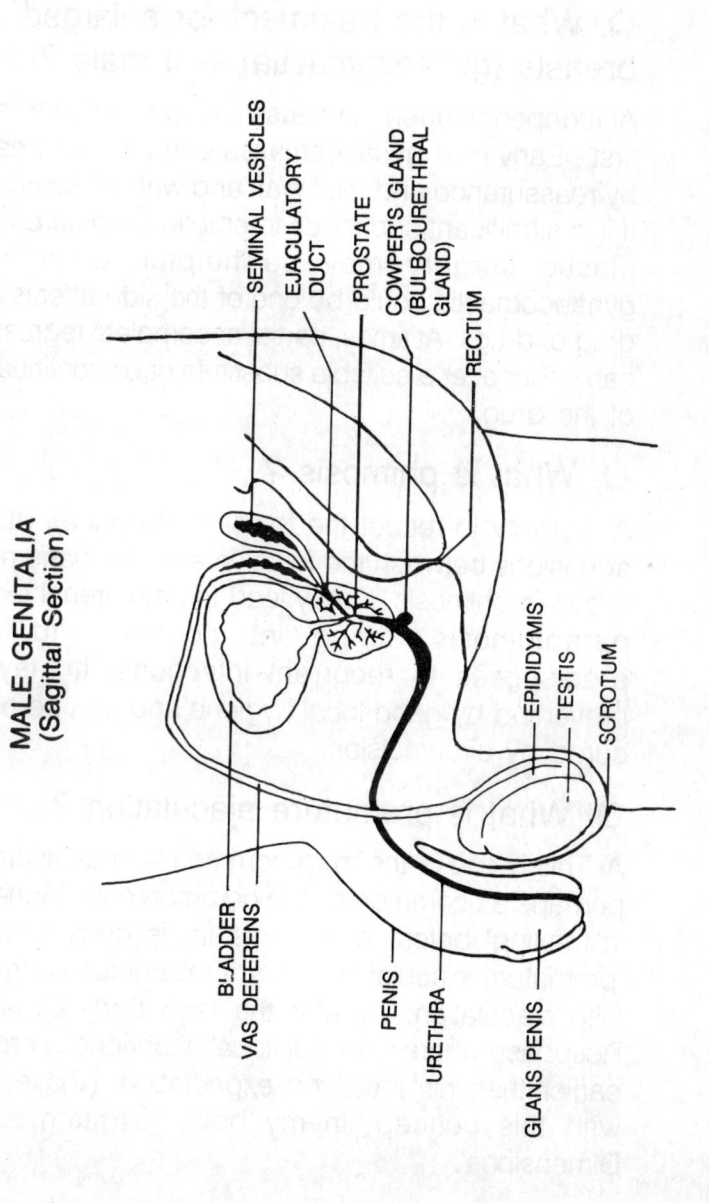

- SEMINAL VESICLES
- EJACULATORY DUCT
- PROSTATE
- COWPER'S GLAND (BULBO-URETHRAL GLAND)
- RECTUM
- EPIDIDYMIS
- TESTIS
- SCROTUM
- BLADDER
- VAS DEFERENS
- PENIS
- URETHRA
- GLANS PENIS

Q. What is the treatment for enlarged breasts (gynaecomastia) in a male ?

A. It depends upon the cause which must be treated first. Early mild gynaecomastia can be best treated by reassurance and the "Wait and watch" approach. If it is significant and leads to emotional disturbance, plastic surgery may be helpful. Sometimes gynaecomastia could be one of the side effects of a drug or drugs. At times, partial or complete regression can occur after a suitable substitute or discontinuation of the drug.

Q. What is phimosis ?

A. Inability to retract the foreskin (prepuce), due to adhesions between the foreskin and the glans penis is called phimosis. It may lead to pain, frenal tear or paraphimosis during intercourse, and also predisposes to recurrent infections. It may be prevented by good local hygiene and can be easily cured by circumcision.

Q. What is premature ejaculation ?

A. This is one of the most common sexual disorders, perhaps as common as the common cold. Generally 'climaxing' before one wants to, is considered as 'premature ejaculation'. This term confuses orgasm with ejaculation. I prefer the term Early Orgasmic Response wherein an individual experiences orgasm earlier than his idealized expectation. I have dealt with this concept in my book 'Orgasm : New Dimensions'.

Q. What are the causes ?

A. The causes may be primary - wherein the disorder exists from the beginning or secondary wherein it occurs subsequent to a prior normal function. The causes and mechanism are as follows:

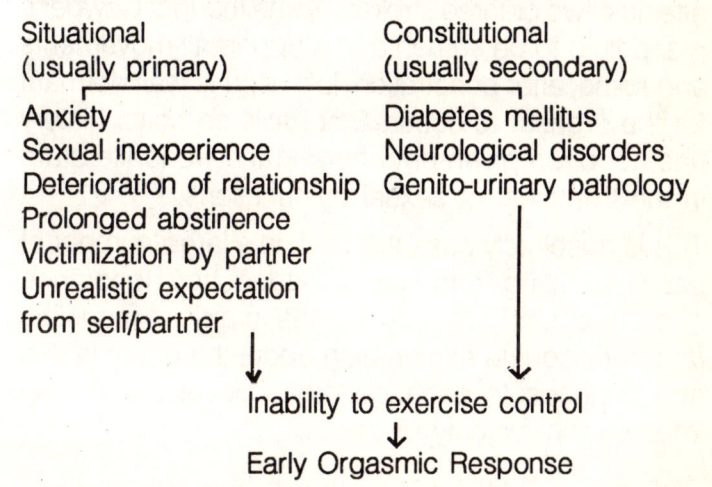

Situational (usually primary)	Constitutional (usually secondary)
Anxiety	Diabetes mellitus
Sexual inexperience	Neurological disorders
Deterioration of relationship	Genito-urinary pathology
Prolonged abstinence	
Victimization by partner	
Unrealistic expectation from self/partner	

↓ ↓

Inability to exercise control
↓
Early Orgasmic Response

Q. What is meant by retarded ejaculation ? Does diabetes have a part to play in cases of retarded ejaculation ?

A. Retarded ejaculation is the opposite of premature ejaculation. Western researchers like Kaplan observe that "undetected diabetes, the most common cryptical physical cause of impotence, may also cause ejaculatory disturbances, but it seems to impair the erectile mechanism more profoundly, or at least equally". In my experience of about 300 cases, which is perhaps the largest in the world to-date, I have not come across a single diabetic. In my series, 50 per cent of the cases of delayed (retarded) ejaculation had inadequate knowledge about the sex act. Some used to move from side to side instead of to and fro; some used to move to and fro but used to pause after just two or three strokes. Some thought Cowper's gland fluid to be semen and stopped all movements and some, after penetration, just used to wait dormant for the orgasm to occur. Emphasis on coital history has not been given anywhere in the world literature in the treatment of sexual dysfunctions.

This is absolutely essential and, in a large number of cases suffering from sexual inadequacy, ignorance about the sex act may be the major responsible factor. Adequate explanation about the act of coitus and methods to enhance orgasmic pleasure may improve the majority of cases.

Q. What is 'orgasmic control' ?

A. In order to understand 'orgasmic control,' it is first necessary to understand the human sexual response. There is an excitement phase where a person is aroused. When he is aroused further, it is known as the plateau phase. This phase is in between excitement and orgasm. In other words, if one wants to have adequate 'orgasmic control', one needs to spend more time in the plateau phase. After this, when the sexual tension heightens further, he reaches a stage which is known as 'orgasmic inevitability'. Once he reaches this point, he will inevitably reach orgasm even if he stops all sensations. One needs to appreciate the feelings and sensations before the sensation of ejaculatory inevitability, as after a split second, there is contraction of the muscles of the pelvic floor and the semen is thrown out in a squirting action.

Note : Sometimes a drop or two of a sticky fluid may come out in the plateau phase. One needs to remember that this is a lubricant and not semen.

Q. How can one improve 'orgasmic control' without a partner ?

A. In order to improve orgasmic control, the following sequence of exercises has proved very effective. They are designed to increase an individual's awareness of sensations and to gradually and progressively develop control. Each step in this exercise may take a week or more.

Ist Step

In this, one masturbates stopping just prior to orgasmic inevitability and allows the arousal to decline. One should continue this 'stop-start' sequence for about 15 minutes. One should pause long enough so as to ensure that one is not back to the stage of orgasmic inevitability when one starts again. The main purpose of this exercise is to learn to recognise the point of orgasmic inevitability and to train oneself to stop stimulation before reaching the point of no return.

2nd Step

After one can comfortably masturbate like this for 15 minutes, some variations can be added.

Change the method of holding the penis in such a way that there is maximum hand contact (folding the hand in the form of vagina). Use oil or lubricant so that the sensations are almost akin to that of the vagina. While doing this, one needs to indulge in fantasies, if any, which one had associated with Early Orgasmic Response. As one enjoys these fantasies he is also preparing himself to avoid Early Orgasmic Response when he is confronted with his partner.

Q. How can one improve 'orgasmic control' with a partner ?

A. One can try similar exercise with the help and co-operation of the partner as follows :-

Stage A - The man lies down on his back allowing the woman to masturbate him, asking her to stop just before he reaches orgasmic inevitability. When the arousal subsides sufficiently, he asks her to start again, repeating the same, for about 15 minutes.

Note: (1) The man should concern himself with his own feelings and should not worry about the partner's sexual needs.

(2) After 15 minutes, the man reaches orgasm, he appreciates and enjoys this sensation.

When he has confidently sustained 15 minutes of stimulation by the partner's hands he can move on to stage B - the second part of the exercise.

Stage B - Here one repeats the above exercise of stage A but instead of allowing him to reach extravaginal orgasm, she stimulates the man to erection and mounts him (female superior position), lowering herself and putting the penis in her vagina. Once the man is inside her, she does not move but remains motionless like a statue. The man gets acquainted with the feeling of the vagina. During this act, if he feels that the orgasm is impending then he tells her and she gets off. Once the feeling subsides he can repeat the same for 15 minutes. After they are able to do this, they can move to stage C.

Stage C - This stage is almost similar to stage B. It is the female above position once again, but this time she moves. The man holds her pelvis and makes her move to and fro. If he feels orgasm is approaching, he stops her movements. Once again, when the feelings recede, he makes her move in a gradual fashion initially so that he does not get stimulated too much and too fast.

One should engage in these exercises until both are quite comfortable with the performance. When one has mastered these three stages, then one can proceed with sexual intercourse in any position.

Q. What is to be done if symptoms recur ?

A. While at any stage of these exercises if you feel you are losing control on your orgasm simply go back to the previous step and work on it for a while until you feel comfortable and confident.

Q. Are there any techniques to delay orgasm ?

A. Many techniques have been used to delay

orgasm. The commonly used ones include mental arithmetic, local anaesthetic ointment, a couple of pegs of alcohol, wearing disposable tissue and a condom around the penis to decrease sensitivity.

Others include :

(1) Voluntarily interrupting and restarting the flow of urine repeatedly (to exercise the pubococcygeus muscle). (2) Taking a deep breath and (voluntarily) contracting the anal sphincter, holding the contraction for 15 to 20 seconds and then releasing. This may be repeated upto 20 times, twice a day. (3) The squeeze technique – (voluntarily) partner squeezes the penis just prior to reaching orgasm.

Q. How does one go about with these exercises ?

A. Identifying the pelvic muscles is simple. Just voluntarily interrupt and restart the flow while passing urine. These are the muscles you need to train. Once identified, try contracting and relaxing these muscles five times, thrice a day; increase it to ten times and then, fifteen and twenty times in subsequent weeks. Continue repetitions thrice a day twenty times for four more weeks. These exercises can be done whilst standing at the bus stop, sitting in the office or at any other time. Dr. Zilbergeld suggests that after contracting the pelvic muscles one should hold them for 3 seconds before relaxation and sixty or seventy of these exercises manoeuvre in a day can lead to sexual benefits in six weeks time.

Q. Are there any exercises which can help male sexuality ?

A. Exercises to strengthen the pelvic muscles, (chiefly those surrounding the penis) help to achieve better control over the orgasmic reflex, improve the quality of orgasm and also increase the circulation of blood in the pelvic area leading to better erectile ability. Better contractions, help in a more complete evacuation of the fluid from the prostate, thus reducing congestion. A pubococcygeus muscle in good tone can provide a firm support to the prostate which helps in reducing prostatic discomfort.

Q. What is the 'squeeze' technique ?

A. In squeeze technique at the time of 'stop' instead

SQUEEZE TECHNIQUE

- URETHRAL MEATUS
- GLANS PENIS
- FRENULUM
- CORONAL RIDGE

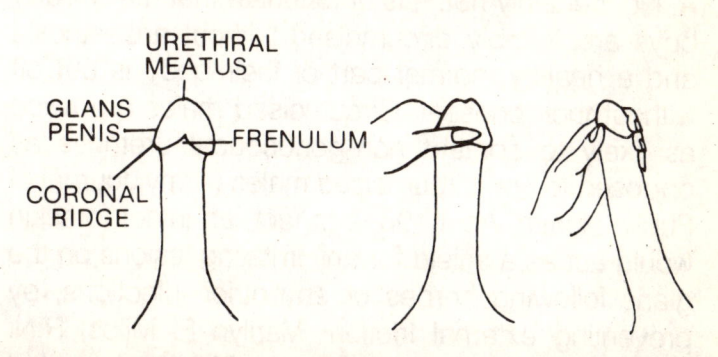

of just taking away the hands from the penis, partner squeezes penis i.e. presses hard for 3 to 4 seconds with the thumb at the frenum and the index and middle fingers on the sides of the coronal ridge.

Q. The technique is so simple, does it really work ?

A. Yes, it does. Though apparently simple in practice the technique is based on a very important concept. It seeks to interrupt an involuntary pleasurable response by introducing a voluntary painful stimulus at the point of inevitability. The supposed 'simplicity' is akin to taking a tablet for some illness. As far as the patient is concerned he is merely taking a tablet. He has no idea about the underlying pharmacological and therapeutic principles involved.

Q. Would you advise circumcision for a new born ?

A. No, certainly not. It is unfortunate that many baby boys are forcibly circumcised without anaesthesia and a healthy, normal part of their body is cut off without their consent. Circumcised males are twice as likely to contact non-gonococcal urethritis as opposed to non-circumcised males (Army Journal of Public Health, April 1987). In fact, an intact foreskin would act as a shield for any irritating lesions on the glans following herpes or any other infections, by preventing external friction. Marilyn F. Milos, R.N. urged in the III World Congress of Victimology that "Health Care providers are obligated, by the ethics of their profession, to discontinue this harmful and unnecessary practice."

The U.S.A. is perhaps the only country in the world in which male infants are at risk for genital surgery without medical or religious reasons. Proper sex education can help eliminate this unnecessary practice.

Q. Do circumcised males have better orgasmic control than non-circumcised ones ?

A. No. This is a myth.

4

FEMALE SEXUALITY

Q. What is virginity ?
A. The word 'virgin' means one who has not had sexual intercourse, which may be verified by an intact hymen. However, a girl whose hymen is intact may have had intercourse; whereas a girl who has never had intercourse may not have an intact hymen. The idea of chastity and virginity needs to be clarified. There are virgin individuals who are not chaste and chaste individuals who are not physiologically virgin.

Q. Is it a fact that girls who menstruate early also tend to begin intercourse early ?

A. No. The timing of coitus depends upon individual sex drive, situational factors and sociocultural background.

Q. Does pre-menstrual tension affect sexuality ?

A. Yes, it does. Women tend to become irritable with associated symptoms such as nausea, backache and breast tenderness. There is a feeling of discomfort in the pelvic region and, at times, there may be emotional disturbances and varying degrees of depression. In some, however, it is found that the sex drive is enhanced, perhaps resulting from increased pelvic congestion, insufficient to cause discomfort but sufficient to cause intense pelvic 'awareness'.

Q. Do oral contraceptive pills prevent pre-menstrual tension ?

A. Yes, oral contraceptive pills do prevent premenstrual tension in about 50% and painful periods in over 90% of the women.

Q. Do women like breast stimulation ?

A. Most women enjoy stimulation of the breasts as they form an important erogenous zone of the female anatomy. But, enjoyment depends upon the way in which they are stimulated. Also there are times when the breasts are tender and an attempt to stimulate them causes pain. This usually occurs premenstrually and during pregnancy and in women using oral contraceptive pills, when the breasts are engorged due to hormonal influence. Hence, it is best to ask the partner about whether "to do, or not to do".

Q. Is the breast size important ?

A. No. Large breasts are not more sensitive to stimulation than smaller one's.

Q. Are there any medicines or creams to enlarge the breasts ?

A. No.

Q. Can the breast size be increased ?

A. Certain exercises can help develop the Pectoralis Major muscles which would add a little bulk to the chest (but not the breasts themselves) and this may help to apparently increase the breast size. Plastic surgery may also prove beneficial.

Q. Are there any exercises for sagging breasts ?

A. There are no exercises which can help sagging breasts because there are no muscles in the breasts except the smooth muscles in the nipple. Wearing of a proper brassiere can help minimise sagging.

Q. Does disparity in breast size require treatment ?

A. Disparity in the size of the breasts may be due to various reasons − physiological and pathological. Disparity due to any pathological cause must be thoroughly investigated and treated. For physiological disparity, no treatment other than counselling and reassurance, is required. For cosmetic reasons, – if the difference is minor, padding the brassiere cup of the smaller breast would suffice. If the difference in size or contour is large then an enhancement/enlargement mammoplasty of the smaller breast or a reduction mammoplasty of the larger one, may be carried out after evaluating each case on individual merit.

Q. Do hair on the breast suggest any pathology ?
A. It is not uncommon for a woman to have a few hair around the areola of the breast which does not need any treatment. However, they may be removed by electrolysis by a qualified person, if one so desires.

Q. Which positions do women prefer ?
A. The best position would depend on the individual's preference and the woman's anatomy. However, in personal interrogation with more than 3,000 women, if given a choice as to which position they would prefer, 75 percentage of them preferred the female superior position. This is perhaps because the clitoris is stimulated better and it also adds a feature of novelty.

Q. Is it necessary to stimulate the clitoris during sexual intercourse ?
A. Some women report that they get enough clitoral stimulation during normal sexual intercourse. Some prefer a little pressure on the clitoris with the pelvic

bone. Some prefer gentle stimulation along with a little pressure. For some women intercourse is enough to reach climax, while for others additional clitoral stimulation is essential.

Q. Do clitoral adhesions lead to inhibited sexual response ?

A. I have yet to come across a case where clitoral adhesions have inhibited sexual response. Besides they are extremely rare.

Q. What is the G-spot and how can one stimulate it ?

A. The G-spot or the Grafenberg spot is an area of increased sensitivity with maximum potential for arousal. It is located on the anterior vaginal wall about two inches from the introitus. After sliding the fingers in that position and with forward, backward or side to side movement, the female will be able to pinpoint the spot where she appreciates increased sensitivity. With increased stimulation, the G-spot swells like a nodule, and becomes firm. Simultaneously clitoral stimulation can enhance sexual pleasure.

Q. What is the most common female sexual problem ?

A. As per my observation, painful sexual intercourse leading to vaginismus is the most common sexual problem.

Q. What could be the cause of excessive vaginal lubrication during sexual intercourse ?

A. Physiologically, lubrication occurs in the vaginal walls during sexual arousal. This could increase in certain conditions of heightened sexual excitement and vaginal infection/allergy. The best thing is to find the cause and treat it. At times, a small dose of an anti-histaminic may prove useful.

Q. Can a virgin become pregnant ?

A. Yes. If the sperms are deposited near the vulva, they may pass through the small hole of an intact hymen and may travel up through the full length of the vagina and uterus and meet the ovum resulting in a pregnancy.

Q. Is sex safe during pregancy ?

A. Usually, a healthy woman can safely indulge in sexual activity during pregnancy. However, coitus should be avoided if there is pain and/or bleeding at any stage. If the woman has aborted in the first three months in the past, coitus during the first trimester should be avoided. In the second trimester coitus is contraindicated if the woman has a history of 'habitual abortion' because the cervical os or the mouth of the uterus is 'incompetent' to hold the foetus. In the last trimester i.e. from the seventh month to labour, one may safely indulge in sexual activity till the day of delivery by altering the position so as to ensure that the direct weight does not fall on the foetus.

It must be understood that whenever, because of any reason, intercourse is forbidden during pregnancy, the woman must avoid reaching orgasm by any other means including masturbation. The contractions of the uterus following masturbation are far more intense as compared to normal sexual intercourse.

An obstetrician may be consulted regarding the indulgence in sexual activity during pregnancy as each case needs to be evaluated individually about any possible contraindication or modification to be made.

Q. Are alcohol and smoking safe during pregnancy ?

A. No, both alcohol and smoking are unsafe during pregnancy as they lead to intrauterine growth retardation.

Q. Can stretch marks on the breasts and abdomen following pregnancy be removed by any medicines ?

A. No. Once stretch marks have occurred, they may somewhat decrease in size on their own but cannot be removed by any medicines or creams. They also occur during puberty, obesity, and Cushing's syndrome besides pregnancy.

Q. When can a woman resume sexual intercourse after delivery ?

A. One should not indulge in sexual intercourse :

(1) If the episiotomy scar (the cut made to ease the birth of the baby) has not healed properly.

(2) If there is bleeding per vaginum.

Usually, after three weeks of delivery a woman can comfortably resume sexual activity.

Q. Is episiotomy necessary during normal delivery ?

A. Yes. It may be advised largely because it facilitates delivery of the fetal head, prevents vaginal and perineal tears, prevents excessive vaginal laxity, and prolapse of the uterus, bladder and rectum.

Q. After pregnancy, many times couples report that they do not experience the pleasure that they used to. Can this be helped ?

A. After normal delivery often vaginal walls become lax and the penovaginal contact reduces. Thus some people do report less pleasure. This can be helped. While doing the episiotomy, the gynaecologist should take one more stitch known as husband's stitch to ensure adequate apposition which helps in increasing the peno-vaginal contact, thus giving more pleasure.

Q. what is the most common cause of lax vagina? How can it be prevented ?

A. This may occur following child birth. It can be best prevented by proper management of labour with perineal support and an adequate and timely episiotomy.

Q. What is the treatment for a lax vagina ?

A. Kegel's exercises for contracting the perineal muscles by holding the urine and releasing it, 20 such contractions and relaxations three times a day, may help increase the muscle tone. If this does not work, one may go in for vaginal reconstructive surgery.

Q. What conditions can make a woman frigid ?

A. Distraction, disturbed interpersonal relationship, anti-hypertensive drugs, tranquilisers sedatives, hypnotics and sometimes oral contraceptives can all lead to decline in sexual desire. Any pain at the time of coitus, whether it is vaginitis, pelvic infection or different uterine position, may lead to frigidity of sudden onset.

Q. What is female circumcision ?

A. It is a barbaric custom of female genital mutilation which varies in the extent of mutilation perpetrated. Its most disfiguring form – the Pharonic circumcision practised in Sudan and Kenya; involves cutting off of the clitoris, labia majora and labia minora followed by close apposition of the tissue that remains leaving only a tiny hole at the bottom for the passage of urine. This severe local mutilation makes sex, a painful encounter. In its mildest form, it involves excision of the clitoris or the clitoral hood alone. It is performed due to the misconception* that unless it is performed a woman will become overtly promiscuous.

Q. Do women ejaculate ?
A. Few women do report squirting of fluid at the time of orgasm, but this is rare. Female ejaculation is an entity which remains to be proven.

Q. What are women's misunderstandings about men's sexuality which may lead to sexual dysfunctions ?
A. Often when a man is a premature ejaculator, many women may consider him a poor lover or the woman may make an attempt to reach orgasm early also. At times, this leads to a shortening of periods of intimacy. In cases of retarded ejaculation, where there is a delay in reaching orgasm, the woman starts getting a feeling that her partner does not love her or she is not attractive to him any more which may disturb the intimate relationship. Also most women consider it improper to actively participate in intercourse and prefer to remain completely passive or only minimally responsive leaving the onus on the male who is now under pressure to perform. This may create a situational anxiety which may impair his response and performance. Even if the male is able to perform properly in these circumstances, the minimal or deliberately subdued response of his partner due to traditional misconceptions will leave him with the feeling that the encounter has not been mutually

---

* *Hanny lightfootklien – First International Conference on Orgasm, 1991* satisfying. If this occurs repeatedly, it instills a sense of inadequacy and frustration in him which may affect his performance and his sex drive may decline.

Q. How should a physician deal with a sexual problem ?

A. After an adequate history taking the physician should try to determine exactly where the problem lies – misconceptions, unrealistic expectations, disturbed interpersonal relaticnships, hostility towards a partner. The physician should counsel the couple as a unit, clarify and explain the situation to them, and clear misconceptions. He may offer specific therapy if and when the situation demands.

5

ORGASM

Q. What is an orgasm ?

A. Orgasm represents the zenith of human pleasurable experiences. 'Orgasm' is derived from the Greek word 'orgaos' which means 'to swell, with lust'. This literal translation very appropriately encompasses the true essence of orgasm.

Orgasm is defined as, 'an explosive cerebrally encoded neuromuscular response, at the peak of sexual arousal by psychobiological stimuli, the pleasurable sensations of which are experienced in association with dispensable pelvic physiological concomitants'.

Q. Why orgasm ?

A. Sex is not merely the means to an end (procreation). It is both, the means to an end, as well as an end in itself (pleasure). Nature, with its natural masterstroke, of providing an inherently sensual pleasure oriented side to our personality, has ingeniously accomplished this dual objective (pleasure + procreation). An attempt to rationalize the philosophy of sex undisputedly establishes the fact that humans indulge in sex to gratify their inherent pleasure instinct. One indulges in sexual activity for what one 'gets' out of it, and not for what one 'may beget' out of it. One indulges, not to 'lose' fluids but to 'gain' an orgasm.

The pleasure principle has, is and always will be 'principal'.

Q. How do you classify orgasmic dysfunctions ?

A. I classify orgasmic dysfunctions, on the basis of one single central parameter – the subjectively reported orgasmic experience, into four broad categories. They represent the discrepancy between one's idealized expectation and one's actual experience.

1. Early Orgasmic Response – (EOR) : This category includes cases in which orgasm is experienced earlier than one's idealized expectations, which are within rational limits.

2. Delayed Orgasmic Response – (DOR) : This category includes cases in which orgasm does ultimately occur, but is delayed beyond one's idealized expectations, which are within rational limits.

3. Impaired Orgasmic Response – (IOR) : This category includes cases in which there is a reduction in the intensity of orgasmic pleasure.

4. Absent Orgasmic Response – (AOR) : This category includes cases in which there is a complete failure to experience orgasmic pleasure.

This classification, based on one central subjective parameter provides conceptual clarity, specific terminologies for different disorders, uniformly encompasses all known male and female disorders, gives information whether a disorder is primary or secondary to some other pathology, and has the scope to include other associated parameters, if and when they are disturbed, alongwith the main diagnosis.

Q. How does one reach orgasm ?

A. When an individual has sexual desire he departs from the normal state and enters into the 'sexual state' and is deemed to have undergone 'sexual grounding'. 'Sexual grounding' or the 'Sexual state' is a state in which the subject becomes receptive to the perception of stimuli inputs as sexual. Once this occurs, psychobiological stimuli arouse the sex centre in the brain which starts sending out impulses, which are usually pleasurable. When such impulses reach the genitalia they lead to congestion of blood which is usually manifested as erection in the male and lubrication in the female. Further stimuli further arouse the individual and eventually lead to orgasm.

MALE SEXUAL RESPONSE

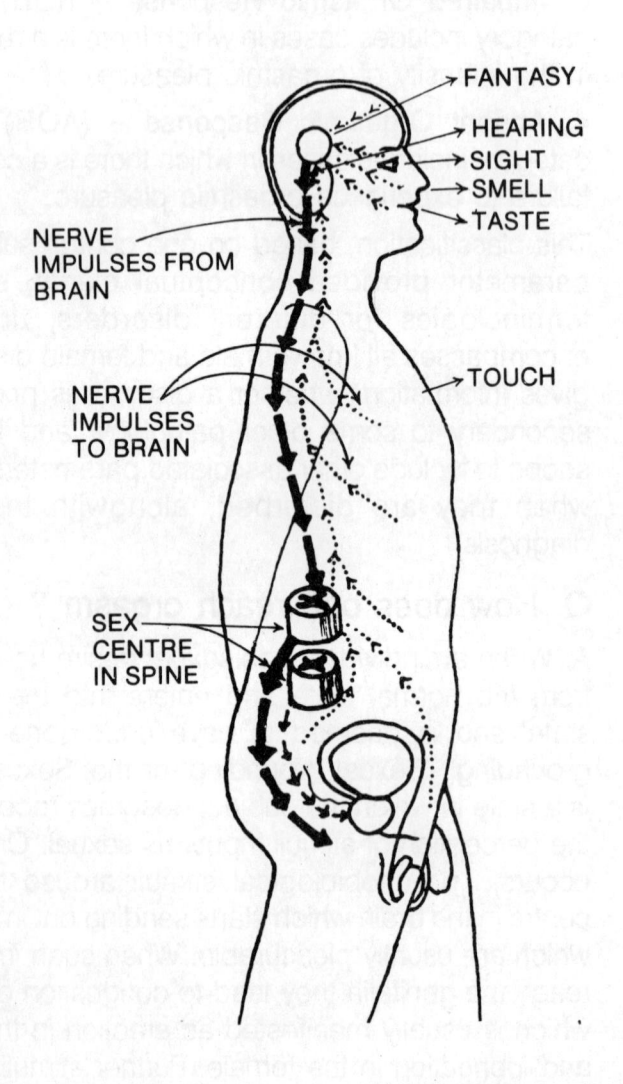

- FANTASY
- HEARING
- SIGHT
- SMELL
- TASTE

NERVE IMPULSES FROM BRAIN

NERVE IMPULSES TO BRAIN

TOUCH

SEX CENTRE IN SPINE

FEMALE SEXUAL RESPONSE

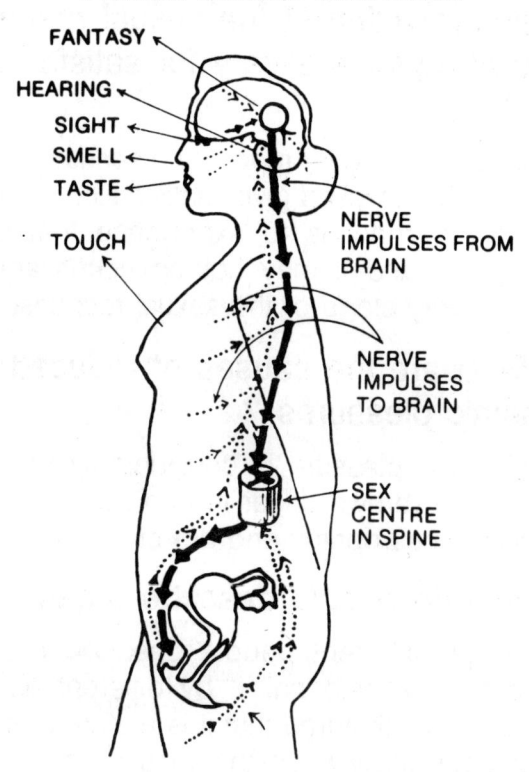

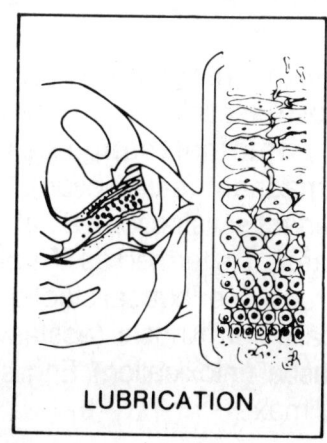

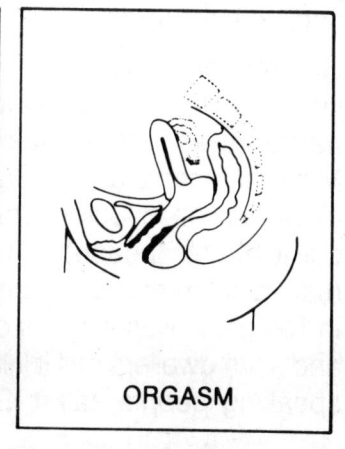

- FANTASY
- HEARING
- SIGHT
- SMELL
- TASTE
- TOUCH

NERVE IMPULSES FROM BRAIN

NERVE IMPULSES TO BRAIN

SEX CENTRE IN SPINE

LUBRICATION

ORGASM

Q. Is completion of the sexual response cycle always necessary for satisfactory sex ?

A. Sex is a method for reaching a sensual objective, which, when achieved gives satisfaction. During sex what is important is to experience that sensual satisfaction, and it may not be necessary to go through every stage of the sexual response cycle.

Q. What are the causes of reduced orgasmic pleasures ?

A. Orgasmic pleasure is considerably reduced in drug abuse (brown sugar in particular), myopathy, alcoholics, neuropathy and anxiety disorders.

Q. How do people describe orgasm ?

A. Though different people describe orgasm in different ways, and call it by different names, in essence they all agree that it is a state of supreme pleasurable satiety where there is a feeling of 'enough and nothing more'.

Gujarati people call it 'Sukh' (happiness), Hindi speakers term it as 'Santosh' (satisfaction) Bohras name it as 'Paramsukh' (eternal happiness), Maharashtrians call it 'Samadhan' (satisfaction), in Urdu it is called 'Sukun' (perfect satisfaction), Sindhis call it 'Shanti' (peace), in Tamil, it is termed as 'Trupti' (satisfaction) and as 'Santrupti' (perfect satisfaction) in Telugu, in Kashmir it is called as 'Khushi' (ecstasy) and slum dwellers call it 'Nasha' (intoxication), English speaking people call it 'Climax'.

It is interesting to note that different people in the diversity of their ethnic, socio-cultural and linguistic backgrounds are united in the expression and description of their orgasmic experience, which they unanimously agree, is, in essence, a sense of supreme pleasurable satiety and ecstasy.

Q. How can one know that one has reached an orgasm ?

A. An orgasm is like a sneeze – it is difficult to describe but once you have had one you know what it feels like. Orgasms may differ. Usually one experiences a heightened sexual ecstasy accompanied by rhythmic vaginal contractions in females and ejaculation in males, followed by a feeling of relaxation.

Q. Are there any physical signs which indicate that an individual has reached climax ?

A. When one reaches orgasm, one usually has gasping uncontrolled movements, or a sense of suspension which are nonverbal communications to the partner that one has had an orgasm. It is usually accompanied by vaginal contractions in female and the visible associate of ejaculation in males. Later, after completion of the sex act, one appears calm and physically satisfied. The signs of having had an orgasm are quite fleeting. The best way is to ask the partner.

Q. Is it normal to reach orgasm by clitoral stimulation ?

A. Absolutely. There are women who are unable to reach climax by vaginal intercourse alone. Climaxing by clitoral stimulation is in no way inferior.

Q. Are different erogenous zones important ?

A. Yes. One need not reach orgasm by genital stimulation alone. One may stimulate any erogenous zone to the point of orgasm.'What is important is the end and not the means to the end'.

Q. Can the use of a diaphragm inhibit a woman's orgasm ?

A. No. The diaphragm fits into the deep portion of the vagina where there are hardly any nerve endings. Real stimulation is in the outer aspect i.e. clitoris and the surrounding area and the outer one-third of the vagina. The diaphragm in no way inhibits a woman's orgasm.

Q. Is it necessary that a woman should reach orgasm during intercourse ?

A. No. It is not necessary that a woman should reach orgasm during intercourse. She may achieve orgasm during foreplay or afterplay by any method including clitoral stimulation. What is important is satisfaction, no matter how one derives it.

Q. Is local genital stimulation absolutely necessary for a woman to reach orgasm?

A. No. Local genital stimulation is not mandatory for reaching orgasm. The female anatomy provides for multiple erogenous zones any of which may be stimulated to reach orgasm. In fact, it has been observed that in the event of absence or trauma to the external genitalia, existing alternate erogenous zones become more sensitive and new ones develop.

Some women can reach orgasm by nipple stimulation alone. I have come across women with absent vaginas who are able to reach orgasm satisfactorily by alternate means.

In a study carried out on ritually circumcised South African women, Hanny Lightfoot Klein reports that these women had retained their orgasmic capacity inspite of the local genital mutilation.

Q. Is there a difference between 'clitoral orgasm' and 'vaginal orgasm'?

A. No, there is no difference. An orgasm may be more or less satisfying depending upon several factors, but whatever be the means of stimulation, ultimately "All roads lead to Rome."

Q. What is multi-orgasm?

A. Multi-orgasm, is experiencing of multiple orgasms one after another, without an intermediate refractory period.

Q. Are males multi-orgasmic ?

A. No. Usually after orgasmic experience, in a male, a refractory period ensues (during which sexual stimuli fail to arouse) following which arousability is regained. Therefore, for multi-orgasmic experience the male has to train himself.

Q. What about females ?

A. Multi-orgasmic capacity is a natural physioanatomical female asset for which no training is required. After experiencing orgasm, females maintain sexual arousability and therefore can experience multiple orgasms in succession. In short, for a female multi-orgasmic capacity is a natural potential and for a male it is an acquired art. ⚥

6

INTERPLAY

Q. What is interplay?
A. Interplay implies the whole spectrum of interaction, that is the entire gamut of motions and emotions, between individuals indulging in 'play'.

Q. Is foreplay important?
A. Yes, extremely important. It kindles desire and marks the beginning of the interplay. An adequate foreplay ensures adequate arousal and promotes sexual compatibility.

Q. Is afterplay important?
A. Yes. Afterplay is as important as foreplay. Though penovaginal sex is regarded as the most intimate

and satisfying form of sexual activity, this is not always true. There are many women who report "I am not worried about orgasm but I would very much appreciate a bit of love play after he is through". *Vatsyayana* in the *Kamasutra*, has given a lot of emphasis to afterplay and he has mentioned that afterplay is equally, if not more, important as foreplay. Most people enjoy being held, cuddled, talked to, and partners need to communicate with each other as to what they prefer. Many-a-time, a woman in her fifties or so would come and report "Doctor, sex is now far more satisfying despite the fact that my husband is unable to achieve erection." Perhaps he is forced to learn or devote more time to foreplay and afterplay which takes away the feeling of mechanical sex and at times when he is unable to perform, there is enough warmth and affection in all forms of sexual activity, the foreplay, the interplay and the afterplay. As mentioned by Dr. Richard J. Cross, "Perhaps the most important part of afterplay is play".

Foreplay introduces and afterplay, summarizes the 'crucial interplay'.

Q. What is the 'normal standard time' for an intercourse ?

A. There is no 'normal standard time' for an intercourse. It depends upon the partners. Intercourse may be continued till it is mutually satisfying. A prolonged intercourse does not necessarily give more pleasure. This is a myth. What is important is not how long ? but how satisfying ?

Q. How often should a couple have sexual intercourse ?

A. Sexual intercourse is the means to an end, the end being pleasure. Therefore, a couple can have intercourse as often as it pleases them. It is a pleasure to be shared between the partners and there is no need to keep a tally. 'Frequent' or 'normal' depends upon the individual couple. The best thing to do is to forget the number's game and indulge as often as it is mutually pleasurable and satisfying. What is important is the quality and not the quantity.

Q. Is frequent intercourse harmful ?

A. Present medical knowledge acknowledges the fact that as long as intercourse occurs among accepting partners and is not associated with physical trauma or irritation, the act itself is not harmful, irrespective of its frequency.

Q. Can one enjoy sex without coitus ?

A. Yes, one can. Sex is not just coitus. It is a total body response! Coitus is one aspect of the whole spectrum of sex.

Q. How ?

A. The most important thing is to communicate to your partner your likes and dislikes. Discuss what both of you like — foreplay, play (intercourse) or afterplay ... at times, this alone will relieve a man and woman from pressure to perform.

One needs to explore the whole body... one might find sucking a woman's nipples a joy for her but often sucking of a man's nipples is more joyful and a pleasant surprise too. Sensuous massaging around the genitals without touching the genitals initially... is greater fun than fondling each other's genitals... if the female is orthodox or inhibited, the male might have to encourage her to talk, to verbalize her feelings and give her feedback about what pleases her and himself the most.

Lubricants sometimes help in enhancing the pleasure. Oral sex could be highly stimulating and satisfying. Men can reach orgasm without erection as well. Some men feel satisfied, and even enjoy giving pleasure to their partners! In reality, coitus is between the two thighs but sex is between the two ears!

Q. How should one find out whether the penis has entered the vagina ?

A. Anatomically there are three openings – urethra, vagina and anus. The urethra is too small; even the little finger cannot go in. The anus is too low. The only place left in between is the vagina. I always advise my about-to-be married male patients to avoid the visual tic-tac-toe between the penis and the vagina and instead, after a little foreplay when they feel an erection coming to leave it to the wife to guide the penis because, after all, she knows her anatomy best and will know where it should go. Though penetration usually takes place easily, it is best to ask the female.

Q. Does reading erotic literature help ?

A. Erotic stories can lead to better sexual arousal. I have come across many couples reading a passage aloud as one of the variations in foreplay and they reported that it had a wonderful effect!

Q. Is fantasizing about other partners during coitus a common phenomenon ?

A. Yes, indulgence in fantasies about one's ideal lovers, ideal love situations etc. during coitus is common. Individuals indulging in this practice claim that it increases sexual arousal.

Q. Are such fantasies harmful ?

A. No, sexual fantasies are not usually harmful. They are nothing to be afraid of or ashamed of. In fact, they enhance sexual arousal making sex life more pleasurable and are often used in therapy. Only if there is an associated guilt, it will create situational anxiety affecting one's response and performance.

Q. Why are some women unable to reach climax during intercourse ?

A. Inadequate foreplay, improper arousal by the partner, male's pressure for coital orgasm, woman's shyness to verbalise the kind of stimulation she needs and her excessive concern to please the partner are the common causes of inability to reach climax during coitus. However, drugs impairing the sexual response, guilt, anxiety and depression, and lax pelvic muscles, may also be responsible for inability to reach climax.

Q. What is the treatment for semen seeping out of the vagina after intercourse ?

A. This is normal and does not require any treatment.

Q. What is vaginismus ?

A. Vaginismus is a condition where there is spasm (severe contraction) of the outer one third of the vagina during an attempt, or anticipation of an attempt, of sexual intercourse, thereby making penetration of the penis impossible.

Q. How is it treated ?

A. It can be easily treated by education, counselling supportive psychotherapy and behaviour modification. No drug or surgery is required.

Q. What are the reasons for pain in the vagina at the time of intercourse (dyspareunia) ?

A. Most often, when the woman is not properly aroused (lubricated) and if the man makes an attempt to enter, it leads to irritation and pain at the time of intercourse. If the pain is always present at the time of intercourse then it could be because of hymenal obstruction, urethral disorders or congenital malformation of the vulva or vagina. It could also occur following post-operative scars and atrophic vulvo-vaginitis (common in menopausal years). If the pain is present occasionally, then one may look for some local infection and/or allergy.

FEMALE GENITALIA

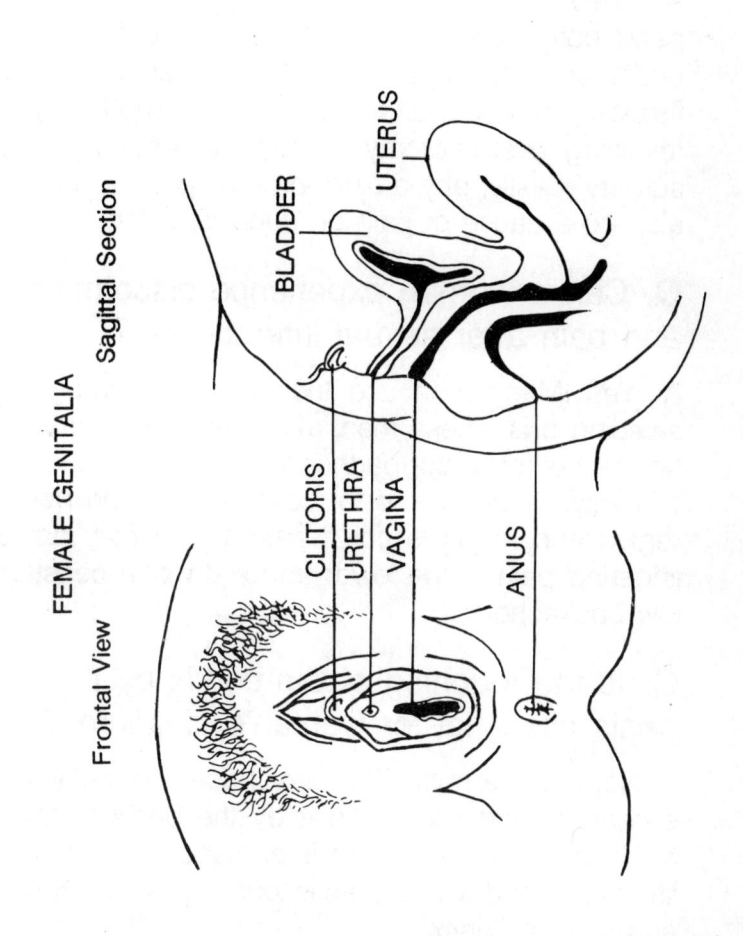

Frontal View — **Sagittal Section**

CLITORIS
URETHRA
VAGINA
ANUS

BLADDER
UTERUS

Q. What are the causes of pain on deep thrusting ?

A. Deep thrust dyspareunia could be because of pelvic congestion, inflammatory disease of the pelvis, endometriosis, lower bowel disease, anal fissures, fistulae, certain ovarian pathologies, short vagina following hysterectomy or vaginal reconstructive surgery. Lastly, any anxiety-provoking situation can also be a cause of pain on deep thrusting.

Q. Can a woman experience discomfort and pain after sexual intercourse ?

A. Yes. Many men use their partners simply as sleeping pills. These men, after they reach orgasm, do not bother about partner satisfaction. She is left half way. There is a lot of congestion in the pelvic region and if this is not released, she may get a lingering pain in the lower abdomen or a constant low backache.

Q. Is the touching of the cervix by the penis essential for woman's pleasure ?

A. No, this is a myth. The cervix does not relay any sensation hence touching it by the penis is futile. Moreover, when a woman is aroused, her uterus is lifted up... and what a man is touching is the sacrum and not the cervix.

Q. Are there different sexual positions ?

A. Yes. Human anatomy allows freedom for innumerable different conjugal positions, any of which

MALE & FEMALE GENITALS IN COITUS

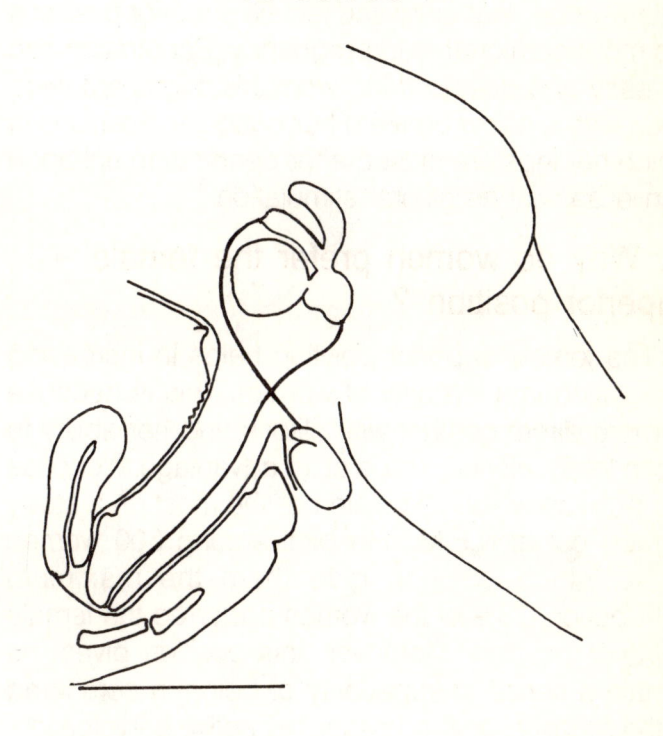

may be used depending on the practicability, and one's individual anatomy and preference.

Q. Are they useful ?
A. Yes. Different positions offer different advantages in different situations with respect to accommodation, penetration and enhancement of pleasure. They also

add a feature of novelty. In addition, a position like female superior is often helpful in delaying the male's climax. It helps in reducing performance anxiety. Side-by-side, rear entry and female superior positions are more comfortable in pregnancy. Penetration can be easy and deeper if the woman's thighs are wide open with a pillow beneath her buttocks. Positions in which her legs are closed after penetration enhance penile as well as clitoral stimulation.

Q. Why do women prefer the female superior position ?

A. The female superior position helps in increasing stimulation in a majority of women. This is because of more direct contact with clitoris and her ability to move freely. Hence, she is at an advantage to choose the position which stimulate her the most. In a study carried out at K.E.M.. Hospital among 500 women as to which position give them the maximum satisfaction, 75% of the women preferred the female superior position. Moreover, this position gives the female a sense of superiority of being in command of the situation, and increases her active participation, thus enhancing arousal.

Q. Which positions are comfortable for the woman during intercourse in late pregnancy ?

The female superior position is more comfortable for a majority of couples. The couple can also try the lateral positions with both anterior and posterior approaches.

Q. Is oral sex normal?

A. Yes. Oral sex can be an excellent variation.

Q. Why do some couples prefer anal sex?

A. Due to the similarity in the neurological innervation of the vagina and anal canal, the central neurological perception is likely to be almost similar in both, vaginal and anal sex. Further, the latter position allows freer access for manual stimulation of the breasts and clitoris. Some experience a better grip whereas others enjoy the novelty. Thus anal sex may be preferred for any one of a multitude of reasons.

ALTERNATIVE ORIENTATIONS

Q. What is an alternative orientation ?
A. Any sexual orientation apart from the popular heterosexual* orientation may be termed as an alternative orientation. It is not necessarily an aberrant or deviant expression of one's sexuality. No one knows definitely why some people develop such alternate preferences.

Q. What is homosexuality ?
A. Sexual attraction towards, and/or indulgence in sexual activity with partners of the same biological

---
* Attraction towards, and/or indulgence in sexual activity with, partners of only the biologically opposite sex.

sex as oneself is called as homosexuality.

Q. Do casual homosexual encounters in early years make an individual a life-long homosexual ?

A. No, they do not. In fact, in a study carried out by Alfred Kinsey, 28 per cent of the females and 50 per cent of the males have had homosexual experiences one time or another in their lives.

Q. Is homosexuality common in India ?

A. Surprisingly, homosexuality in India is far more common than thought of. Male homosexuality, female homosexuality and bisexuality are on the increase in India today.

Q. What is lesbianism ?

A. Mutual sexual attraction, and/or indulgence in sexual activity between two women is termed as lesbianism. It is a specific term for female homosexuality.

Q. What is bisexuality ?

A. Attraction towards, and/or indulgence in sexual activity with partners of both biological sexes is termed as bisexuality.

Q. What health hazards does bisexuality pose ?

A. Bisexuals are usually more promiscuous and are prone to health hazards due to multiple sexual partners such as STD's, AIDS, rectal prolapse with sphincter incontinence. They are also more prone to paraphilias.

Q. What is Paraphilia ?

A. "Para" means 'beyond', and "philia" means love. This includes Fetishism, Transvestism, Zoophilia, Pedophilia, Exhibitionism, Voyeurism, Sexual Masochism, Sexual Sadism, and others. They are more common in males than among females.

Fetishism : the condition in which a person is dependent on a talisman or fetish object, substance, or part of the body in order to obtain erotic arousal and facilitate or achieve orgasm.

Transvestism : behaviourally, the act of dressing in the clothes of the opposite sex; psychically, the condition of feeling compelled to cross-dress, often in relation to sexual arousal and attainment of orgasm.

Zoophilia : the condition of being responsive to, or depending on, sexual activity with an animal in order to obtain erotic arousal and facilitate orgasm; also known as bestiality. Sexual contact (oral or genital) with an animal may occur sporadically in the course of human development without leading to long-term zoophilia.

Pedophilia : the condition in which an adult is responsive or dependent on the imagery or actuality of erotic/sexual activity with a pre-pubertal or early pubertal boy or girl, in order to obtain erotic arousal and facilitate or achieve orgasm. A pedophiliac may be a male or a female. Pedophilic activity may be replayed in fantasy during masturbation or copulation with an older partner.

Exhibitionism : the condition of being responsive to or dependent on the surprise, debasement, shock, or outcry of stranger (usually female) unexpectedly exposed to the sight of the genitals, in order to obtain one's erotic arousal and facilitate or achieve orgasm. The actual event may be replayed in a masturbation or coital fantasy.

Voyeurism : It is also called as scoptophilia. The desire to observe the genital of others or to watch sexual intercourse becomes the condition of erotic excitement and gratification. A voyeur is also known as a "peeping Tom." The actual event may be replayed in a masturbation or a coital fantasy.

Masochism : the condition of being responsive to or being dependent on receiving punishment and humiliation in order to obtain erotic arousal and facilitate or achieve orgasm. As the partner of a sadist, a person may impersonate a masochist for commercial gain, within the limits set by the pain threshold.

Sadism : the condition of being responsive to or dependent on punishing or humiliating one's partner in order to obtain erotic arousal and facilitates orgasm. A person, especially a woman, may impersonate a sadist to oblige masochistic partners for commercial gain.

Frottage : rubbing or pressing against some object, usually the buttocks of a fully clothed woman, in public places, becomes the condition for sexual excitement.

Gerontophilia: the condition in which one prefers to obtain sexual gratification from an elderly person.

Necrophilia: in this condition, gratification is obtained by indulging in sexual activity with a corpse.

Q. What is the difference between a transvestite and a transsexual ?

A. A transvestite is an individual who becomes sexually aroused by donning the apparel of the opposite sex, and a transsexual is one who strongly feels that he or she belongs to the opposite sex.

Q. How can one diagnose transsexualism ?

A. Transsexualism is an overriding feeling of discomfort with one's anatomic sex and a constant desire to be rid of one's genitals to become a member of the opposite sex. In other words, a male mind in a female's body and vice versa. The diagnosis is made only if the disturbance has been continuous for at least two years; if there is no evidence of psychological disorder like schizophrenia; and is not associated with physical intersex or genetic abnormality. The differential diagnosis must be made among true transsexualism, transvestism and homosexuality. Physician should be aware that Gender transposition may occur in cases of severe personality disorganisation associated with psychosis. A behavioural sex change may emerge even later in life in certain rare cases of temporal lobe epilepsy or as a consequence of senile dementia.

Q. Are eunuchs transsexuals ?

A. No. Eunuchs are not necessarily transsexuals. They are castrated males, who have had their testicles removed prior to puberty so that the secondary sexual characters do not develop. As against this, transsexuals are individuals who have an overwhelming desire to be the opposite sex. ⚥

8

OLD AGE

Q. What are the common sexual misconceptions prevalent among the middle aged men and women ?

A. Men harbour the misconception that increasing age and excessive use may lead to weakening of the genitals and end in 'seminal bankruptcy'. Because of this misguided belief, they observe sexual abstinence. One should remember that it is disuse which leads to atrophy and not the use. As a man grows older, he walks slow, he talks slow but he expects that his erection should not be slow! One needs to remember that this is a normal phenomenon. Some are under the impression that "one failure in making it means an end to sex life". As a result, many men move from effective sexual functioning to various degrees of impotence. I always emphasize that occasional failures are common and failure does not mean an end. Women harbour the misconception that menopause marks the end of sex life. Menopause merely marks the end of a woman's reproductive career and not the conjugal career which can continue upto the end of one's biological life. In fact, the maturity of the partner's and the relationship, alongwith guaranteed natural contraception may enhance the sex life. The misconception that "sex after 60 is not possible" needs to be changed. Men and women can continue to remain sexually active till the last day of their lives provided they are in sound physical and mental health.

Q. What physical changes occur when a person grows older ?

A. As a man grows older, erection takes a longer time to occur. Similarly, in women, lubrication takes a longer time to occur. A man may often require direct physical stimulation to achieve erection and the same is also true of a woman's lubrication. The colour of the semen changes from white to light yellow, the consistency gets thinner and the quantity decreases. When, people are not informed about these facts, anxiety can be generated, as there is a vast discrepancy between the unrealistic expectations and the real experience. This paralyses the sexual response leading to avoidance of sexual overtures. Older persons tend to become obese because of sedentary lives, lack of exercise and changes in hormonal levels. Exercises for toning up the muscles and good functioning of the body, are essential. All these help in improving the self-image and making a better sex life.

Q. Can a very active sex life in the early years affect one's sexual life later ?

A. A very active sexual life in youth does not precipitate an early termination of the sex drive or capacity. On the contrary, persons having a strong sexual interest and capacity in the early years are more likely to retain the same in the later years. This was confirmed by a longitudinal study on sexual behaviour and old age.

Q. What are the most common conditions which could decrease sex drive in later years ?

A. The common reasons for a reduced sex drive in later years are :
1. Monotony and loss of interest
2. Changes in physical appearance
3. Misconceptions about one's waning sexuality
4. Lack of communication
5. Depression

Q. How does one overcome depression ?

A. Supportive psychotherapy could be of great help and if the depression is severe then a psychiatrist's intervention may be helpful.

Q. Does female sexual desire increase or decrease at menopause ?

A. Some women report an increase while others report a decrease in sexual desire at menopause. Increase in sexual desire may be because of relative freedom from pregnancy and hence one may respond and perform with greater abandon and enthusiasm. Some women harbour the misconception that menopause marks the end of their sexual career and this fear (about their waning sexuality) increases their sex drive so that they may reaffirm their femininity. A decline in sexual desire could be because of physical reasons. During menopause (or even a few years earlier), a reduction in the secretion of the ovarian hormones may cause atrophy of the vaginal epithelium which leads to reduction in lubrication and hence pain at the time of sexual intercourse (which can be remedied by estrogen replacement therapy). This causes a decline in sexual desire and a woman avoids sexual overtures. Depression and anxiety are common features and they also tend to reduce the sexual desire.

Q. Is taking of estrogens at menopause safe?

A. It is advisable to consult your doctor, prior to the use of hormonal preparations during menopause. Estrogen replacement can avoid atrophic vaginitis which leads to painful intercourse, and also helps in preventing osteoporosis which usually leads to frequent fractures. It would be best to take estrogen with progesterone in monthly cycles. It may also help in menopausal depression.

Q. Does Benign prostatic hyperplasia (BPH) cause increased libido in the later years?

A. No. It does not cause increased libido.

Q. What is the physician's role in helping patients with sexual problems in later years?

A. The physician should explain to both partners, the physiological changes that occur with age and reassure them that a healthy conjugal relationship is a normal and acceptable form of behaviour, at any age, because sexuality is as important for the old as it is for the young. Sex education material may be provided to educate the couple, clear any misconceptions and desensitize previous taboos. Sensate focus exercises (sensuous interplay short of intercourse), or other alternatives such as oral sex, more foreplay, different positions may be advised depending upon the individual needs.

ILL HEALTH

Q. What are the most common sexual dysfunctions among diabetics ?

A. Sexual dysfunction is common amongst diabetics. The causes could be vascular, neurological or psychological. In diabetic impotence, the history is suggestive of presence of desire but decline in erectile ability at all times. Usually the onset of the problem is gradual. In some, the presenting symptom could be premature ejaculation and rarely retrograde ejaculation. Diabetic women sometimes complain of reduction in lubrication and difficulty in reaching orgasm. Monilial infection may further reduce lubrication and associated itching makes intercourse uncomfortable. Monilial infection, often leads to Balanitis. A misconception that "all diabetics become impotent" may itself lead to psychogenic sexual dysfunction.

Q. Is sex after heart disease safe ?

A. One must consult a cardiologist, because what is good for one person is not necessarily good for another. Hellerstein and Friedman have studied cardio-pulmonary responses in middle-aged middle-class convalescent males engaging in sexual activity with their wives in the privacy of their bedrooms. From their studies it was concluded that if a cardiac patient could walk on a treadmill at 3 miles per hour asymptomatically and without undue elevation of blood pressure or electrocardiographic changes, he could safely perform sexual activity.

Q. What limits should one observe ?

A. There is nothing like a limit in sex; either you indulge or you do not. The incidence of heart attacks during sexual activity, as per statistics, is 1 in 200. This could have happened even otherwise like while passing urine or going to the toilet. However, the best person to advise you would be a cardiologist because the patient's regimen needs to be tailored according to individual needs.

The following precautions may be useful :

(1) Avoid clandestine sexual activity as it tends to increase the heart rate even more than usual

(2) Avoid elaborate meals and alcohol prior to the

sex act as a lot of energy and blood flow is being utilized for digestion

(3) It is preferable to have sexual intercourse in the morning when one is not fatigued

(4) It is advisable to do regular physical exercise so that sexual exercise need not be an unaccustomed exertion

(5) One may keep a nitroglycerine tablet handy or use nitroglycerine ointment if anticipating chest pain.

Q. Is the female superior position helpful ?

A. No. It is a myth derived by common sense. Scientific research has proved that alteration in sexual positions such as the man taking the bottom position and a passive role has no particular energy saving advantage. The blood pressure and heart rates have been directly measured and are found to be the same in men in the male superior as well as the female superior positions.

Q. Has blood pressure anything to do with sex ?

A. There is a marked increase in blood pressure during sexual intercourse. Theoretically speaking, very high blood pressure does pose a danger of cerebral haemorrhage and myocardial infarction. A study recently conducted clearly showed that cerebral haemorrhage among patients with high blood pressure occurred as frequently during sleep and defaecation as during sexual intercourse. However, it is desirable to control high blood pressure. Patients need to be informed very clearly that the danger of catastrophic events is negligible with the short term changes that occur during intercourse and other physical activities. It is equally if not more, important, to inform the patients about the likely side effects of anti-hypertensive drugs on sexual response.

Q. Which anti-hypertensive medicines have the least sexual side effects ?

A. No generalisation can be made. However, diuretics and vasodilators have the least sexual side effects. Yoga and Transcendental Meditation with biofeedback could be a safe adjunct.

Q. "Whatever anti-hypertensive medications I use, my sex desire and potency get reduced considerably... What should I do — reduce the dose, stop the drug or stop sex ?"

A. Consult a competent physician. On most occasions, the medication can be changed to a drug which has the same effect on the target symptom, without paralysing the sexual system.

Q. What precautions should one take during coitus if one is suffering from bronchial asthma ?

A. The sex act is not very stressful. Shortness of

breath is a natural response during the sex act and more so if one has an acute episode of bronchial asthma. It becomes more intense if anxiety is accompanied. Use of a bronchodilator prior to sexual activity could be helpful.

Q. What sexual problems can a man with kidney failure have ?

A. He may have less desire and inadequate erection due to anaemia, uraemia and testicular dysfunction. These lead to low testosterone production. Psychological problems like depression leading to decline in sexual desire are common. Anxiety is another common feature where sexual arousal becomes difficult.

Q. What is Peyronie's disease ?

A. This is a condition usually found in men who are in their fifties and above. There is development of a fibrous plaque in the penis leading to curvature apparent during erection. It may cause discomfort and, at times, pain during intercourse. Usually, this is a self limiting disease and no treatment is needed. Operative procedures are rarely resorted to and a drug named Potaba is often used in the treatment.

Q. What are the causes of blood in semen ?

A. Any condition which can give rise to congestion and inflammation of the prostate and seminal vesicles can cause blood in semen. Trauma and urethritis may also lead to blood in semen.

Q. Can hepatitis (jaundice) lead to sexual problems?

A. Yes, it kills appetite for sex. In addition, the fear of transmitting or acquiring the disease via sexual contact adds anxiety to the existing problem.

Q. Can one indulge in sexual intercourse during hepatitis?

A. This will depend upon the cause and the type of hepatitis. If it is of the non-infectious type, one may safely indulge in sexual activity. If it is due to a viral infection, then it is transmissible to the partner and one should take certain precautions.

Q. What precautions should be taken?

A. Viral hepatitis can be transmitted through the patient's sputum, saliva, semen, blood and other body secretions. Faeces are also highly contaminated with this virus. As the genital area may be contaminated with faeces, it is advisable to clean the private parts properly and avoid any sexual activity which involves exchange of body fluids. If one does indulge in sexual activity then a condom must be used for whatever protection it affords, as it prevents an exchange of coital secretions.

Q. How does arthritis affect sexual relationships?

A. In arthritis, pain and mechanical discomfort of the joints usually leads to disturbance in the sex act, especially where there is an involvement of hip, knees or back. Factors like frustration, anger, dependency and low self image due to deformity, lead to depression. Steroid side effects like obesity and moon like face complement this.

Q. What are the treatment options available ?

A. Discussion with the partner about alternatives and more comfortable positions is the best option. Speak to the partner about the areas which arouse you the most and inform him/her about the painful areas. Plan your drug schedule in such a way that you take pain relievers prior to the sex act. Select the best time for coitus i.e. osteoarthritis is worst in the evening and better in the morning and the reverse is true for rheumatoid arthritis. This will make the sexual encounter more comfortable. A shower or a tub bath together with warm water, will act as a good foreplay activity, in addition to diminishing stiffness and pain. Use of lubricants can enhance the pleasure. It is particularly useful in Sjogren's syndrome, where along with reduction of other secretions of the body, there is reduction in vaginal lubrication. Advice will vary with individual cases.

Q. Which sexual position would be better for an individual who has localised low back pain ?

A. Low back pain could occur because of lumbago, disc lesion or arthritis. The affected partner should lie on his/her back with the hips flexed. In this position, the psoas muscles are relaxed and hence the vertebral column remains flat on the bed, which is more comfortable as compared to the superior position.

Q. Can a man have sexual intercourse after a prostate operation ?

A. Yes, he can. Currently the greatest number of prostatectomies are done via the trans-urethral route. The quality of erection remains the same at the time of climax and the men experiences the same pleasure. The ejaculation usually remains unaffected though in some individuals the quantity of ejaculate outside may be less or absent because of retrograde ejaculation. In younger patients ejaculation can be preserved even better by doing newer procedures such as balloon dilatation and microwave therapy.

Q. What is the effect of a (radical) mastectomy on a woman's sexuality ?

A. Though anatomically mutilating, theoretically a radical mastectomy should have no effect on a woman's sexuality as her physiology remains unchanged. However, the physical mutilation may wreak a similar psychological trauma with a great effect on a woman's self image and self esteem. She may begin to harbour the feeling that she has become less feminine and hence less attractive. This may depress her and make her withdraw from social and sexual contacts. The surgeon must explain to the patient the operative procedure, the intra-operative risks, the possible outcome and that it is being performed as a potentially life saving curative procedure. To patients who are very apprehensive about the disfigurement he may explain that reconstructive mammoplasty can be performed if so desired.

Q. Can a person lead a normal sex life after hysterectomy ?

A. Yes. Women who were sexually active before hysterectomy continue to be sexually active after surgery. Sexual life remains unchanged, as the coital function is preserved. Hysterectomy usually involves the removal of the uterus but if it necessitates removal of the ovaries as well, then the patient may require estrogen supplementation therapy.

Q. Is there any relation between sex and obesity ?

A. On the face of it, sex and obesity may have no connection at all. Often sexual inadequacy may lead to anxiety and depression which may result in increased food intake in some individuals. Hormonal disturbances may also lead to obesity. This may produce interference with normal sexual functioning and overall sluggish behaviour. Sedentary habits and lack of exercise are common in obese individuals. This may result in flabby muscles and sexual pleasure may decrease as the specific muscles that play a part in love-making get easily fatigued.

Q. Can smoking hinder sexual response ?

A. Smoking does lead to constriction of the blood

vessels leading to inadequate supply of blood to the genital organs which may lead to sexual inadequacy. Discontinuance of smoking for a heavy smoker leads to increase in desire and many report better erectile ability also.

Q. Do routine X-rays induce impotence ?
A. No.

Q. What are the causes of decline in sexual desire ?
A. The desire could decline situationally because of several reasons like dislike of partner, his/her body odour, his/her behaviour, disturbed interpersonal relationship, any bereavement, loss, stress, disappointments or sexual incompatibility. It may also decline if there is fear of pregnancy or sexually transmitted diseases. The lowering of desire could be due to depression or schizophrenia. Constitutional disorders responsible for decline in sexual desire could be due to testicular or ovarian pathology, liver pathology etc. The desire may also decline owing to other endocrine disturbances and drugs like antihypertensive, psychotropic, cimetidine and certain Ayurvedic preparations.

Q. When is sexual desire excessive ?
A. The term 'excess' needs to be defined. In our culture, increased male sexual activity is considered as a sign of masculinity, while the same behaviour in a woman is considered to be a stigma or an

illness, e.g. nymphomania. Increased desire can be seen in mania where there is acceleration of activity in all spheres. Sometimes, there is increased sexual desire in schizophrenic patients, perhaps because of loss of inhibitions. Organic diseases, like a tumour in the frontal lobe of the brain, disturbances following head injuries or the period after an epileptic attack, may be associated with increased sexual desire.

MARRIAGE

What is a marriage ?

According to Hindu philosophy marriage in Sanskrit means 'lagna' i.e. union. A marriage is, ideally, a close or intimate association or union. It is not merely the legal or religious formalization of a social institution.

Q. Is sex important in a marriage ?

A. Yes, it is an important, albeit, a small part of the marital relationship. Love is more important... Erich Fromm mentions "Sexual desire is, in the minds of most people, coupled with the idea of love; they are easily misled to conclude that they love each other when they want each other physically. To love somebody is not just a strong feeling. It is a decision, a judgement, a promise."

Q. What are the most common sexual complaints amongst spouses ? why ?

A. The most common complaint is of sexual dissatisfaction with one's spouse. This is usually because of a communication gap. Perhaps, the partners have never asked each other their likes, dislikes and preferences, due to shyness. Inadequate foreplay is common problem. Verbal, visual as well as tactile foreplay constitute a healthy sensual interlude for a mutually satisfying interplay. One may be unaware that there are more erogenous zones apart from the genitalia which may be stimulated to enhance pleasure. During the act of love, one must communicate one's love to one's partner and ex-communicate everything else. There is no place for a communication gap which if present, would bring discord to a healthy marital relationship.

Q. What are the common causes of marital stress amongst middle aged couples ?

A. Middle aged couples often have a stressed relationship. The enthusiasm of the initial years has decreased. One's mind is preoccupied with other matters which are considered more important. The man, becomes more devoted to his career, to ensure the financial security of his family. His spouse too, is devoted to the pursuit of her household and maternal duties. However, though there is a communication gap attraction is still present. This is a critical period of the marriage and, if nurtured carefully could mature into a warm companionship. Each partner must be understanding of the others duties and responsibilities and try to adjust accordingly. They should make a conscious effort to ensure that the quality of the time they spend together compensates for the diminished quantity.

Q. Why do people have extramarital affairs?

A. People have extramarital affairs for several reasons. Sometimes it is dullness or monotony and lack of adequate sexual response from the partner which motivates an individual to go in for an extramarital affair. Sometimes, it is an individual's personality which inclines him towards this sort of behaviour. Often change, experiment and adventure are the motives for one's indulgence in extramarital affairs. Lack of love and emotional involvement too may lead to extramarital affairs. Truly, it has been said by Benjamin Franklin "where there is a marriage without love, there will be love without marriage."

Q. Do you recommend extramarital affairs?

A. I neither recommend nor condemn them. A good counsellor should not impose his own values on his clients.

Q. Is masturbation after marriage normal ?

A. Yes. Masturbation is normal even in married individuals. It may be encouraged during periods of separation, illnesses and in conditions where one partner's sexual needs cannot be coped with by the other.

Q. How can one overcome boredom in a disturbed marital harmony ?

A. It is essential that the partners accept the fact that the problem exists and for which both have to share equal responsibility. Just talking about it, at times, could be helpful. Taking a vacation leading to a change of environment may be a wonderful experience. Having sex at the same time, in the same manner, at the same place, gives a tinge of monotony and dullness. Sometimes, experimenting with new sensual and sexual approaches, reading sexual materials, seeing erotic pictures and movies, love-play with no pressure to perform, can have a therapeutic effect in a couple's physical relationship. Making love somewhere other than the bed; creating a sensual atmosphere with music, candle light and the use of a mirror; watching your own reflection help as psychological aphrodisiacs. Taking a bath together, using scented body oils and the use of a vibrator, can help dissolve bedroom boredom and enhance pleasure. Poor communication between the partners a common cause for boredom has to be remedied. Romance need not end with marriage. Romance rejuvenates passion, making one's sex life more interesting. Just sending flowers on birthdays and anniversaries or giving a kiss while leaving the house is not enough. At times, caressing your partner's particular part may give her the feeling that you are still attracted to her. Going out on a rainy evening or taking an unscheduled weekend off for no particular reason, help in rekindling excitement in love making. Sex alone is merely a physical thing but pleasure in sex has emotional as well as intellectual dimensions. The importance of romantic social interplay and sensual interplay along with sexual interplay cannot be overemphasized.

Q. What sexual problems do doctors face ?

A. The problems are the same as with other people. However, because of the work situations, as a physician serves society at the expense of his role as a husband and father, he may have already strained relationship with his family. At times, the problems are worse because there is reluctance on the part of the physician to seek marital help. Divorce is not only damaging but also tarnishes the social image. All these lead to deterioration in the relationship in general, and the sexual relationship, in particular.

Q. What are the effects of favourable work situations on the sexual life of professionals ?

A. Success and profound work satisfaction or a deeper involvement in a job or profession can also give rise to sexual problems. For example, if work is pleasurable and enjoyable, one gets more involved in work and dislike going back home. In a situation like this, they merely do their 'duty' at home by giving token love and affection to their spouse and children, but their heart is in their work. Sometimes, it so happens that they are already disenchanted with those at home and dream about their 'favourite objects' at work. Deceitful and clandestine meetings also compel a professional to find fault with those at home and glorify the love objects with whom pleasures can be shared leaving 'pain' at home.

Q. What are the effects of adverse work situations on the sexual life of professionals ?

A. Sexual problems among professionals in India and abroad are most often accompanied by anxiety. This particular anxiety in our country is again born out of myths and misconceptions. One of the most common misconceptions, is "One failure in 'making it' is the end of sex life". Strangely enough, problems during work are carried into the bedroom. Sometimes, anger and resentment arising out of behaviour of seniors or co-workers can be projected onto one's partner, making the spouse an unacceptable mate. Hostility and resentment can create situations which cannot easily be forgotten at bed time even with the help of drugs and dopes. When one is under stress, it is difficult to seduce or arouse him. Relaxation seems impossible. All these lead to difficulties in sexual performance.

FAMILY PLANNING

Q. Why is Family Planning necessary today?

A. Population control assumes importance if one considers the fact that forty years ago the population of our country was a mere three hundred and forty million which, in 1981 had swelled to six hundred and seventy million, in 1991, increased to eight hundred and forty four million and, by the turn of the century, may well escalate to the one billion mark! This galloping increase has to be tackled on a war footing. The socio-economic benefits of family planning to the individual, society and nation cannot be overemphasized. One needs to remember that 'Family Planning' is 'Family Welfare'.

Q. What are the different contraceptive methods available today ?

A. Today, wide range of contraceptive methods are available and the current approach is to provide a 'cafeteria choice' i.e. to offer all the different methods to an individual, from which, any method may be adopted depending on individual suitability and preference.

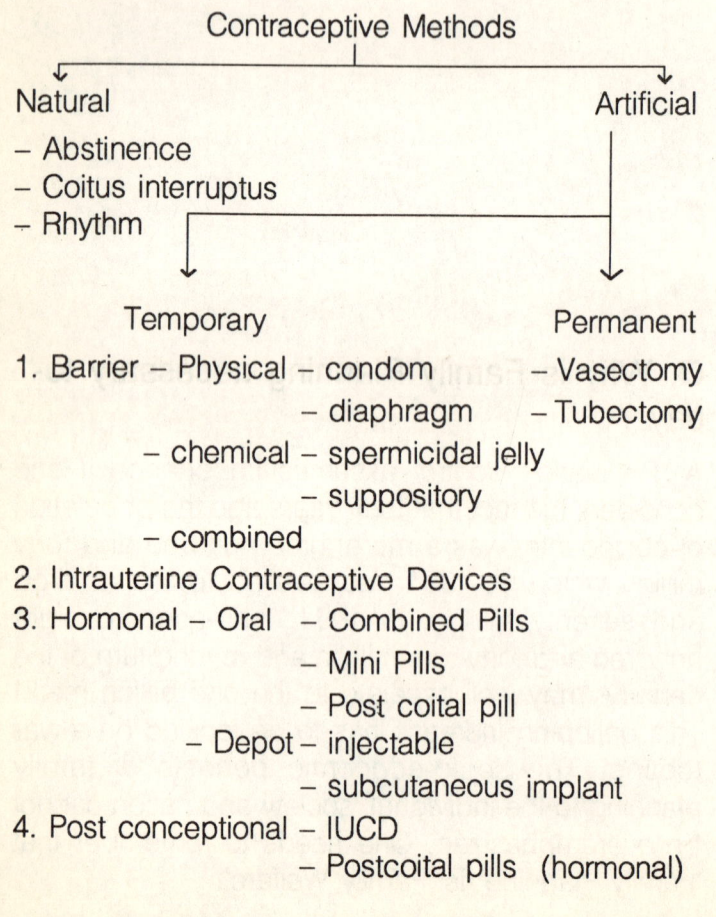

```
                    Contraceptive Methods
                    ↓                   ↓
              Natural              Artificial
              - Abstinence
              - Coitus interruptus
              - Rhythm
                          ↓                    ↓
                     Temporary             Permanent
```

1. Barrier – Physical – condom   – Vasectomy
                     – diaphragm   – Tubectomy
            – chemical – spermicidal jelly
                      – suppository
            – combined
2. Intrauterine Contraceptive Devices
3. Hormonal – Oral   – Combined Pills
                     – Mini Pills
                     – Post coital pill
            – Depot – injectable
                    – subcutaneous implant
4. Post conceptional – IUCD
                    – Postcoital pills (hormonal)

Q. Is vaginal douche after intercourse a safe method of contraception ?

A. No. It is practised as a method of local hygiene and not as a method of contraception.

Q. Is coitus interruptus a safe method of contraception ?

A. No. Coitus interruptus involves withdrawal of the penis just prior to ejaculation so that ejaculation occurs extravaginally. It requires repeated motivation and a tremendous amount of will-power, during each act of coitus, to be effective. Hence, the failure rate is very high. Moreover, some men may not be able to predict the moment of inevitability everytime. It also affects the response and performance as the individual is constantly under tension to withdraw at the moment of inevitability and is unable to enjoy the intimacy. This gives a tinge of mechanical sex and often leaves the partner unsatisfied.

Q. How should a condom be used ?

A. Though seemingly simple, a certain protocol needs to be followed when using a condom for contraception :

1. A new condom should be used for every act of coitus.
2. Condoms are available in pre-tested, pre-sterilized packs and need not be tested prior to use.
3. It is to be rolled onto the erect penis just prior to insertion. The practice of delaying and putting it

on just before ejaculation should be avoided.

4. It should be removed immediately after ejaculation otherwise the penis becomes flaccid and the semen is likely to spill into the vagina.
5. For removal, it is to be held on to the base of the penis, and should be withdrawn along with the penis.
6. It may be used with some spermicidal jelly to maximise its contraceptive effect.

Q. How do contraceptive (spermicidal) suppositories work ?

A. They work by immobilizing the sperm by chemical actions and need to be inserted at least 5 minutes prior to intercourse. The effect lasts for an hour and usually gives protection for a single coitus. If she desires to indulge in intercourse again, she will need another suppository. Some of them are biodegradable and need not be removed after use. Instructions regarding use should be very clear and lucid. There are instances of women who have used spermicidal suppositories orally and some who have inserted them in the anus! It is best to use them under the guidance of a gynaecologist.

Q. What is an intrauterine contraceptive device (IUCD) ?

A. It is a contraceptive device which has to be inserted into the uterus.

There are medicated and non-medicated varieties

available. The advantages include: the one time motivation, no systemic metabolic side effects, no interference with local sensitivity, high success rate and long duration of action. The disadvantages include increased incidence of pelvic inflammatory disease, increased bleeding, dysmenorrhoea and increased risk of ectopic pregnancy.

Q. What are the contraindications for using an intrauterine contraceptive device (IUCD) ?

A. IUCD should not be used if a woman has menorrhagia (excessive bleeding), an abnormal uterine cavity; undiagnosed bleeding from the uterus or the vagina; pelvic infection; history of ectopic pregnancy or tubal surgery. IUCD is generally not advised for women who have not yet borne a child.

Q. What are the common misconceptions about 'the pill' ?

A. There are women who are under the mistaken impression that the effect of the pill lingers for many months after they have discontinued it and may lead to sterility. Some, again mistakenly, believe that for effective contraception a pill should be taken after each coitus while others discontinue taking the pill just because of vague symptoms of mimicking pregnancy.

Q. Are oral contraceptive pills effective from the first cycle ?

A. Oral contraceptive pills act by interrupting the ovulation (release of the egg), thus creating an anovulatory cycle. It takes at least one 'pill cycle' for anovulation to get established. Hence, during the first cycle, one must use an alternative method of contraception.

Q. What should a woman do if she forgets to take a pill ?

A. If the woman forgets to take the pill at the usual time and remembers the lapse on the same day, she should take the scheduled pill on the same day, as soon as she remembers it. If the woman forgets to take 'the pill' for one day and remembers so only on the next day, she should take two pills on that day i.e. the 'forgotten pill' of the previous day, in addition to the scheduled pill for the day.

If, however there is a lapse in taking pills for two consecutive days then the woman must consider herself 'unprotected' and adopt another method of contraception for the rest of the cycle.

Q. When are oral contraceptive pills contraindicated ?

A. If the woman has a history of liver disease, abnormal liver function tests, steroid dependent cancer e.g. breast cancer, abnormal uterine/vaginal bleeding or evidence of circulatory disease including hypertension, migraine; oral contraceptive pills are contraindicated. Other contraindications include, diabetes, the first six months in the case of nursing mothers and epilepsy. However, a gynaecologist's opinion should be sought prior to use.

Q. What is post coital contraception ?

A. Post coital contraception is the employment of a contraceptive measure after intercourse, within 48 to 72 hours of an unprotected intercourse. It is more effective when used within 24 hours.

1. Hormonal – This involves taking high doses of an estrogen (Diethyl stilboesterol – 25-50 mg/day for five days or ethinyl estradiol 0.5-5mg/day for five days) and is associated with high incidence of nausea and vomiting.

Alternatively two tablets of a combination pill (ethinyl estradiol 100 micro gm and 0.5 mg levonorgestrel taken initially, followed by two more tablets after precisely twelve hours, can be given. If this type of contraceptive fails there is risk of foetal malformation.

2. IUCD – A simpler method is to introduce an IUCD, if acceptable, especially a copper containing device.

Q. What is vasectomy ?

A. Vasectomy is a permanent method of contraception by male sterilization. It is performed under local anaesthesia. Two small one cm incisions are made on either side of the scrotum. This gives

VASECTOMY

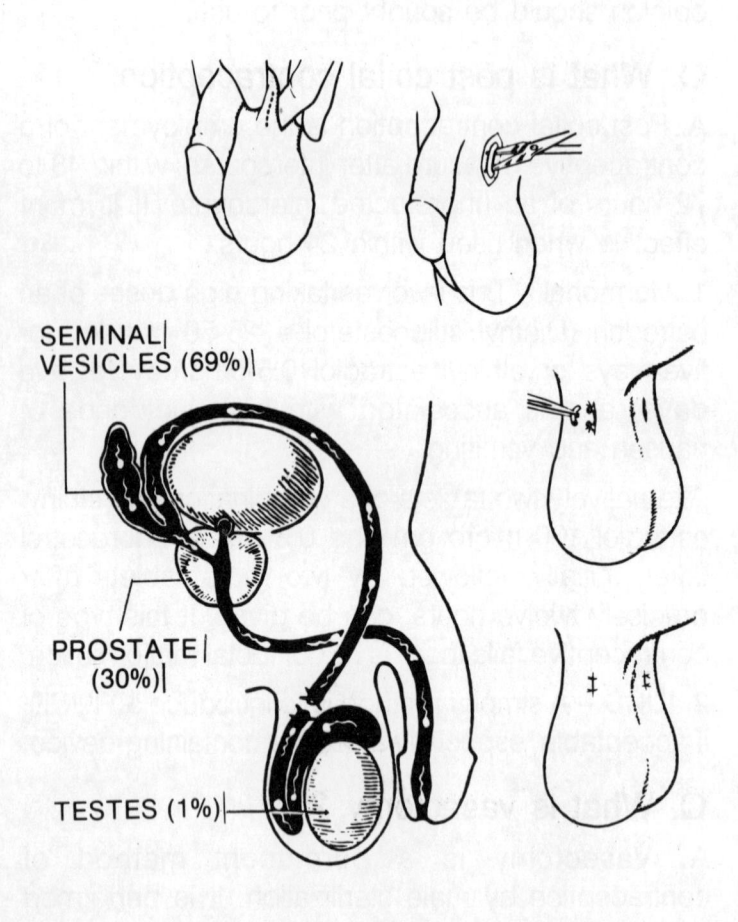

SEMINAL VESICLES (69%)

PROSTATE (30%)

TESTES (1%)

access to the spermatic cord in which the vas is found. A small segment (one cm) of the vas is cut and the snipped ends are tied (closed) off, so that the sperm will be unable to pass through. The incisions are then closed with an absorbable suture. This operation is simpler than the sterilization of a female. Hospitalisation is not necessary and the patient can walk back home. The procedure only affects the fertility and the virility is left intact.

Q. In which conditions, vasectomy should not be encouraged ?

A. Vasectomy should be postponed in cases where
(1) a man is equating his masculinity with fathering of the child,
(2) there are unresolved doubts and conflicts about the procedure and its outcome,
(3) Local conditions where surgery becomes difficult (infection, varicocele, large hydrocele, inguinal hernia, filariasis or scar tissue from surgery).

Vasectomy should be deferred until a specialist is consulted.

Q. Are there any complications after vasectomy ?

A. Yes, occasionally. They may be surgical, immunological or psychological. Surgical complications are the least serious. They consist of bleeding (scrotal haematoma) or infection. This usually occurs a week later.

Immunological complications are extremely rare and no cause and effect relationship is known. Psychological complications occur chiefly because of inadequate counselling prior to the operation.

Q. What precautions should one take after vasectomy to prevent surgical complications ?

A. An athletic supporter or a tight fitting jockey type underwear should be worn for a week to help relieve swelling and to support the scrotum to relieve the discomfort. The small gauze bandages protecting the incisions should be changed every two days.

Q. What happens to the residual sperms ?

A. The residual spermatozoa are phagocytosed (swallowed and destroyed) by the lymphatics of the testicle and epididymis and are rapidly disposed off.

Q. Does the male hormone (testosterone) level go down after vasectomy ?

A. No. Vasectomy has no effect on testosterone levels. A study was carried out by my colleagues and myself at the Institute of Research in Reproduction (ICMR), Bombay, on 45 vasectomised males with sexual dysfunctions. The duration of vasectomy was from fourteen days to fourteen years and revealed no significant change in the testosterone levels.

Q. Is sexual desire and potency affected by vasectomy ?

A. No. The testes have two variety of cells. One variety secrete testosterone which goes directly into the blood stream and is responsible for sexual desire and potency. The sperms are produced by the other variety of cells and they pass through a tube known as the vas. Thus, tying or ligation of the vas will have no effect on desire or potency. Sex life will remain unchanged. Erections, ejaculations and pleasure at orgasm will be as before.

Q. Can vasectomy help sexual functioning ?

A. By removing the fear of possible pregnancy and eliminating the need for artificial aids which often impair local sensitivity, vasectomy may lead to an improvement in the sexual performance in some individuals.

Q. How soon after vasectomy can one resume sexual activity without contraception ?

A. Don't count days, count the number of ejaculations. At least 10 ejaculations after vasectomy and/or two consecutive semen analysis reports need to be sperm negative. Till then, effective contraceptive methods should be used.

Q. Is vasectomy reversible ?

A. Yes, but the success of the reversal operation depends upon the skill of the surgeon, the technique used at the time of sterilization, duration after which reanastomosis is performed and the technique used for reanastomosis. However even after a successful reversal operation by the best of micro-surgical techniques, a man's chances of impregnating the female are fifty-fifty.

Q. How can vasectomy be made more acceptable ?

A. Ideally, the man and his wife both should be counselled together about the surgical procedure, the operative risk and the outcome. It needs to be emphasized to the couple that the procedure is merely contraceptive and will have no effect on the man's virility. Ligating the vas will not have any effect on sexual desire, response and performance. The orgasmic capacity, ejaculation and quantity of ejaculate all remain the same. This will remove any misconceptions that the couple may harbour about the procedure. Its advantages over other methods of contraception, such as its permanency, high success rate, only one time motivation required, absence of systemic side effects, non-impairment of local sensitivity, potential reversibility and its relative ease and safety over tubectomy should also be stressed additionally. Thus, vasectomy can be made more acceptable by education.

Q. What is tubectomy?

A. Tubectomy is a permanent method of contraception by female sterilization, involving the ligation and excision of the tubes to interrupt the passage of ova. Its contraceptive measure does not leave any residual effect on the female's sexuality.

Q. Is tubectomy reversible?

A. Yes. Tubectomy is reversible by microsurgical techniques, but, this is more difficult than reversal of vasectomy. The success rate depends upon the method of tubectomy and the skill of operating surgeon.

Q. Does tubectomy affect estrogen levels?

A. No. Ligation of the tubes merely interrupts the passage of the ova thus preventing conception. It leaves the hormonal levels unchanged and has no effect on the female sexual desire.

Q. Is there any change in sexual enjoyment after tubectomy?

A. In fact, it may enhance one's sexuality as it offers contraception without decreasing local sensitivity, unlike barrier contraceptives.

Q. Does the female superior position prevent pregnancy?

A. Alas! No!

12

APHRODISIACS

Q. What is an aphrodisiac (sex tonics) ?

A. 'Aphrodisiacs' are foods, herbs, potions, or drugs which are believed to increase sexual desire and improve sexual performance. Aphrodisiacs are named after the Greek Goddess of love 'Aphrodite' who emerged from the sea when the God Chronos killed his father and threw his genitals into the sea (which probably accounts for the popularity of sea foods as aphrodisiacs). The mythical belief in foods and drugs to stimulate one's sexuality is a delusion as old as the human race. Different aphrodisiacs have been in vogue at different times. Recently in the 1960s, an oriental herb called 'ginseng' was very popular. The root of this plant became the largest selling aphrodisiac in the American market. In the 1970s, **'royal jelly'** became a popular energizer for the gonads. Later on, Vitamin E and zinc became the most commonly accepted nutritional aphrodisiacs. It is interesting to note that most of these 'aphrodisiacs' remotely resemble the genitals which probably accounts for their 'efficacy' – the belief being known as the 'Doctrine of Signatures'.

Q. How do aphrodisiacs work ?

A. Sex tonics usually 'work' in three ways. Some like alcohol, marijuana, alter the mental state; others increase the flow of blood in the genital apparatus e.g. yohimbine, and some cause severe irritation and inflammation of the genito-urinary tract e.g. spanish fly. Sex tonics as such have no effect on sexuality. The most effective mode of action is the well-known mechanism of suggestion. In my opinion, if a tablet is given, it is the picture of a horse on the cover that works, not the tablet; if an injection is given, by and large it is the prick of the needle that works and not the contents of the syringe! The fact is that no food or drug on earth to-day is direct sex stimulant.

Q. What is the effect of alcohol on sexual functioning ?

A. Alcohol is essentially a central nervous system depressant. In small doses it gives a feeling of warmth and well being and removes social inhibitions which probably accounts for its popularity as an 'aphrodisiac'. However, as mentioned by

SEX TONICS
(Mechanism of Action)

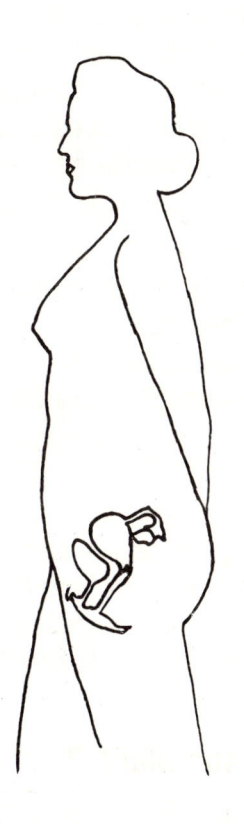

PLACEBO

ALTERING MENTAL STATE

INCREASING FLOW OF BLOOD

IRRITATING MUCOSAL PASSAGE

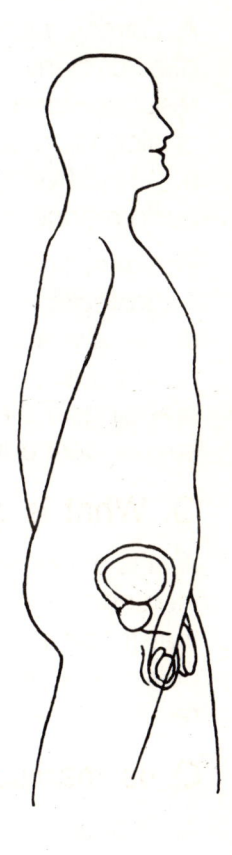

Shakespeare, "The desire it provoketh, but taketh away the performance" is unfortunately, but undisputedly, true.

Q. What are the long term effects of alcohol on an individual's sexual functioning ?

A. Chronic alcoholism impairs the sexual functioning due to many causes. The repeated impairment of response and performance during acute episodes of alcohol intake create anxiety which proves to be a 'psychological barrier' to response and performance in subsequent sexual encounters also.

Besides, chronic alcoholism, results in hepatic and neurologic damage. This leads to decreased sensitivity and impotence in the male and early menopause, excessive menstrual and intermenstrual bleeding in the female and an overall decrease in sexual desire in both sexes.

Q. What is ginseng ?

A. It is a root from Panax ginseng – a perennial herb indigenous to East Asia. Recent research reveals that it has no beneficial effect on sexual desire or potency. Its reputed aphrodisiac effect is due to the resemblance of its root to the phallus.

Q. Is marijuana a sexual stimulant ?

A. Though its use has been extensive all over the world, the use of marijuana as an aphrodisiac is undependable and the effects are largely because of reduction of inhibition, increased suggestibility and time distortion effect.

Q. What are the sexual effects of cocaine?

A. It leads to temporary sexual excitability but with flight of ideas, fear reactions and paranoid thinking.

Q. Is vitamin E a sex tonic?

A. The myth, "vitamin E — a sex tonic", perhaps came from a study done on rats in the 1960s and 1970s. Rats deficient in vitamin E were found to have sex-organ problems. When vitamin E was given to the rats, some of the problems were alleviated and on this basis it might have been concluded that vitamin E could not only correct these deficiencies in human beings but would also actually improve sexual functioning. Research was conducted in the U.S.A. in 1979 and it revealed that vitamin E led to no improvement in sexual arousal or behaviour.

Q. What is testosterone?

A. Testosterone is the natural androgen produced by the Leydig cells of the testes in men. If the cells do not function, puberty is delayed and sexual infantilism persists. If these cells fail later in life after puberty, a man experiences loss of libido and potency, a reduced ejaculate, a gradual decrease in testicular size and slow growing facial hair.

Q. What is your opinion about testosterone in the treatment of sexual dysfunctions ?

A. Testosterone is often used for its 'supposed' aphrodisiac effect. However, it is seldom effective and is useful only in those exceptional cases where there is a genuine lack of testosterone in the body or where there is evidence of failure in the development of secondary sexual characteristics or in old age when there is evidence of low levels of testosterone. If used irrationally in young individuals, it may cause decrease in sperm count. Abnormal liver functions and cases of liver malignancy have also been reported. If administered in females, hirsutism, male pattern baldness, enlargement of the clitoris and deepening of the voice are the chief side effects. Abnormalities of glucose tolerance curve (test for diabetes) may be encountered and disturbances could occur in previously stable diabetes. It is often used, empirically, to improve sexual desire and performance in middle aged men. However, significant decrease in testosterone secretion in middle aged men is very uncommon.

When using testosterone in the elderly it is advisable to do a rectal examination prior to its use, as it may precipitate occult or microscopic cancer of the prostate gland. Unless the symptoms and metabolic investigations reveal decrease in testosterone levels, it should never be used.

Q. What is papaverine ?

A. Papaverine is a drug that acts as a vasodilator and muscle relaxant. Direct injection of the drug into the penis will result in a firm and long lasting erection.

Q. Are there any side effects of using papaverine ?

A. Sometimes the erection achieved by papaverine injection fails to subside. Hence, it should be used with caution. One should avoid using papaverine more than twice in a week, as it may lead to scarring, bruising etc. Long term use may cause fibrosis and curvature of the penis. The drug also has the disadvantage of losing its effectiveness over a period of time. It should be used only under physician's guidance.

Q. What is your opinion about the expensive *paan* sold in some metropolitan cities as a sex tonic ?

A. It is a common practice among some about-to-be married grooms, to take a *paan* called *palang tod* (cot-breaker) on the wedding night to ensure a good (manly!) performance. This *paan* contains drugs and makes a man feel tremendously drowsy. There is also an associated effect of time distortion. A minute's performance may make him feel as if he has performed for an hour. This *paan* does more harm than good.

Q. Have you ever prescribed a sex tonic?

A. Just once. A few years ago, a client from a mideastern country was referred to me. After I treated him for his problem, he insisted that I write down a prescription for a sex tonic. I refused. Then the referring physician told me that the patient was obsessed by his failing potency and begged me to at least prescribe a vitamin pill. I was furious, but I decided to prescribe a sort of baby food and told him to take one spoonful three times a day. After six months, he called back to say that he was fine. In fact, he felt so good about his sex life he asked me if he could continue his doses of baby food every day. That was the first and, will probably be, the last time that I ever prescribed, or will prescribe, a sex tonic.

Q. What is the best natural aphrodisiac?

A. The best natural aphrodisiac is an attractive partner passionately asking to be enjoyed. The 'ideal' aphrodisiac still eludes us, but the quest for it continues, as hope springs eternal.

AIDS

Q. What is AIDS ?

A. It is an Acquired Immune Deficiency Syndrome, a viral disease in which the immune system becomes so weak that the individual becomes susceptible to any infection or disease that an otherwise healthy person would be able to resist easily. AIDS victims can be devastated by the common cold or by a simple attack of diarrhoea.

Q. Do we need to worry about AIDS ?

A. Yes. AIDS can spread easily through any infected secretion of an AIDS patient. So far no cure has been discovered for this eventually fatal disease which cripples the immune system making the body increasingly prone to infections. Once contracted the prognosis is usually poor, and the motto one must follow is "Prevention is the only Cure."

Q. Is AIDS contagious ?

A. Yes. The AIDS virus has been transmitted between male homosexuals, heterosexuals, intravenous drug users sharing contaminated needles, from blood transfusions, contaminated blood products, contaminated secretions like saliva, semen, tears, urine of an infected person, as well as vertical transmission from mother to infant. One can also get infected by tattooing, shaving, dental work, acupuncture, electrolysis needle, surgical procedures etc. if sterile aseptic precautions are not used.

Q. Why is anal sex more risky than vaginal sex ?

A. The rectal mucosa is more prone to abrasions and tears as compared to the vaginal mucosa. Thus, a discontinuity of the lining mucosa creates a direct portal of entry into the blood stream. Thus, AIDS virus from an infected partner will be transmitted more easily during anal sex.

Q. What precautions should a homosexual take ?

A. If possible, avoid. If not, then while indulging in oral sex, avoid taking the partner's semen in your mouth. While having anal sex insist on the partner wearing a condom.

Q. Can one tell by inspecting a potential partner if he/she is infected ?

A. No. One cannot definitely say whether an individual harbours the virus by mere inspection, as the vast majority of individuals who have been infected are 'Symptomless carriers' and show no evidence whatsoever, of the infection. They may themselves be unaware that they are infected. The best method of finding out whether an individual is infected, is to undergo a blood test.

Q. What precautions can one take to avoid AIDS through sexual contact ?

A. As mentioned earlier with a potentially infected partner "prevention is the only cure". However, precautions that one may take to reduce the risk of transmission are:

1. Avoid sex with individuals who are in a 'high risk' group such as – male and female prostitutes, homosexuals, bisexuals, people with multiple partners, individuals who have had sexual contact with an AIDS patient, hemophiliacs, patients on renal dialysis, intravenous drug abusers etc.
2. Avoid sex with multiple partners especially with unknown/casual partners.
3. Avoid sexual activity which leads to exchange of body fluids as this is risky (the virus has been isolated from the saliva, blood, semen, tears and urine of infected individuals). Therefore avoid oral sex, peno-vaginal sex and peno-rectal sex.

4. Use condoms during sex as they reduce the risk of transmission of the virus.

Q. What are safe sexual practices for uninfected individuals ?

A. Uninfected individuals should avoid all sexual practices which involve exchange of body fluids, when indulging in sexual activity with potentially infected partners. They may safely indulge in non-oral and non-coital sexual practices such as fondling, stimulation of erogenous zones, sensate focus exercises, mutual or self masturbation, penetration alternatives such as intercourse between the thighs, inter mammary intercourse etc. An orgasm is an orgasm, and is equally satisfying by whatever means it is achieved.

Q. What is the ideal thing to prevent AIDS (through sexual transmission) in our country ?

A. In a populous country such as India, it would be ideal to use barrier contraceptive devices like the condom, which may offer protection against infection as well as conception.

Q. How can parents help their children in avoiding AIDS ?

A. Parents should educate their children about AIDS so that when they become sexually active they know exactly what risks they are taking. Just moralising does not help to persuade people in changing their behaviour. It must be emphasised that there is no cure for AIDS; at the same time one should also emphasise that it is not transmitted via casual contacts, like serving meals, giving hair cuts, shaking hands, using public toilets or swimming pools. Early and accurate information is absolutely essential in the prevention of AIDS, as well as, unnecessary panic and anxiety.

TOWARDS HEALTHY SEXUALITY

Q. What is sexual hygiene ?

A. Sexual hygiene involves developing and maintaining a healthy sexuality and preventing sexual dysfunctions.

Q. Is it necessary to clean the private parts daily ?

A. Yes. Ideally, one should clean the private parts daily. This ensures good local hygiene, makes one more aware of and comfortable with one's private parts, removing the misconception that touching the private parts is a taboo, draws early attention to any local pathology and prevent the development of intertriginous skin infections.

A man should clean the parts daily, especially retracting the foreskin upto the base of the glans penis. This prevents the development of phimosis which is a painful condition and may lead to complications like paraphimosis. A woman must wash the vagina in a direction away from vagina and not towards it, to prevent faecal contamination of the vagina and urethra.

Q. Should a virgin use a tampon?

A. The use of tampons in young girls should be encouraged as it affords an opportunity for the young woman to become acquainted with her own sexual anatomy and to overcome any taboos regarding handling her genitals. Moreover, the gradual minimal stretching of the hymenal opening prepares her for later intercourse without difficulty. It would also give the young lady a healthier attitude towards her menstrual period. However, one should realise that the hymen may rupture while using tampons and may cause problems in those who harbour the misconception that a virgin must have an intact hymen!

Q. Should a woman use vaginal douches or deodorants?

A. No. This is not necessary. In fact it may cause irritation and inflammation and may increase the risk of infection by altering the vaginal flora. Often, women use deodorants to mask offensive vaginal odours usually secondary to infection. The root cause must be determined and treated accordingly.

Q. Can one indulge in intercourse during menses ?

A. Certainly. Sex during menstruation is absolutely safe. If both partners so desire, then they can most certainly indulge in it. Menstrual material is physiologic. Many couples find coitus more enjoyable at this time mainly because there is relative freedom from possible pregnancy and also because of the enhanced sensation promoted by a moist vagina.

Many women are under the impression that intercourse during menses may lead to increased bleeding. Women do report heavier bleeding initially but the duration is often shortened considerably and the rhythmic contractions of the uterus help evacuation of the menstrual material more rapidly. In fact, a satisfying sexual intercourse during the menstrual period reduces cramps and alleviates the feeling of heavy discomfort resulting from pelvic congestion.

Note: Some doctors do advise the use of condoms especially in the case of those women who do not keep their perineum clean. Menstrual material may become a rich source of culture medium for the growth of bacteria owing to its close proximity to the anus, and may facilitate an inflammatory reaction in the man's urethra.

Q. What are personal massagers ? Are they useful ?

A. 'Personal massagers' are also known as vibrators. These vibrators can help in providing additional stimulation in some individuals. Some women prefer to hold a vibrator on the clitoris even when rhythmic thrusting of the penis in the vagina is on. Most men prefer to use a vibrator with slow speed on the area around the scrotum, and the underside of the penis. It is particularly helpful in older men as they require more intense physical stimulation as compared to younger men, and a vibrator could serve as a good adjunct.

Q. Which is the best vibrator ?

A. There are several models available, like the plastic battery-operated ones and the electrically-operated ones with multiple attachments. However, one must not forget that at times even a finger could prove to be the best vibrator!

Q. Is testicular self examination (TSE) necessary for an adult male ?

A. Yes. Every adult male should perform the TSE every month. Testicular cancer is one of the most common form of cancers in men between the ages of 20 & 40. If diagnosed early it can be cured completely.

Symptoms and signs :

The first sign of testicular cancer is usually a slight enlargement of one of the testes and a change in consistency. Pain may be absent but often there is a dull ache in the lower abdomen and groin, together with a sensation of dragging and heaviness. These symptoms may be due to some other condition that is readily treated.

How to perform the TSE :

It is a simple three-minute monthly self-examination. The best time is after a warm bath or shower, when the scrotal skin is most relaxed. The following are the simple steps for an effective TSE:

1. Do the TSE first on one testicle, then on the other.
2. Use both hands to examine each testicle.
3. Place your fingers behind your testicle, with the thumb in the front.
4. Roll each testicle gently between the thumb and fingers of both hands. Most likely, the testicles will feel smooth and spongy if they are completely normal. But if you feel any hard lumps or nodules on the front or side of the testicles, you must see your doctor promptly. Only the doctor can make the diagnosis whether it is malignant or not.

The TSE is a healthy habit that should be practised regularly, every month.

Q. Why must one perform breast self examination ? How ?

A. Almost all breast cancers are first detected by women themselves. Detection of breast cancer in the early stages, when it is localized, is of paramount importance, because if treated properly, the disease can be cured completely. Hence, the importance of self examination of the breasts, monthly, as a routine health habit to be practised by all women over the age of 20 years. It should be performed at about the

Fig. 1

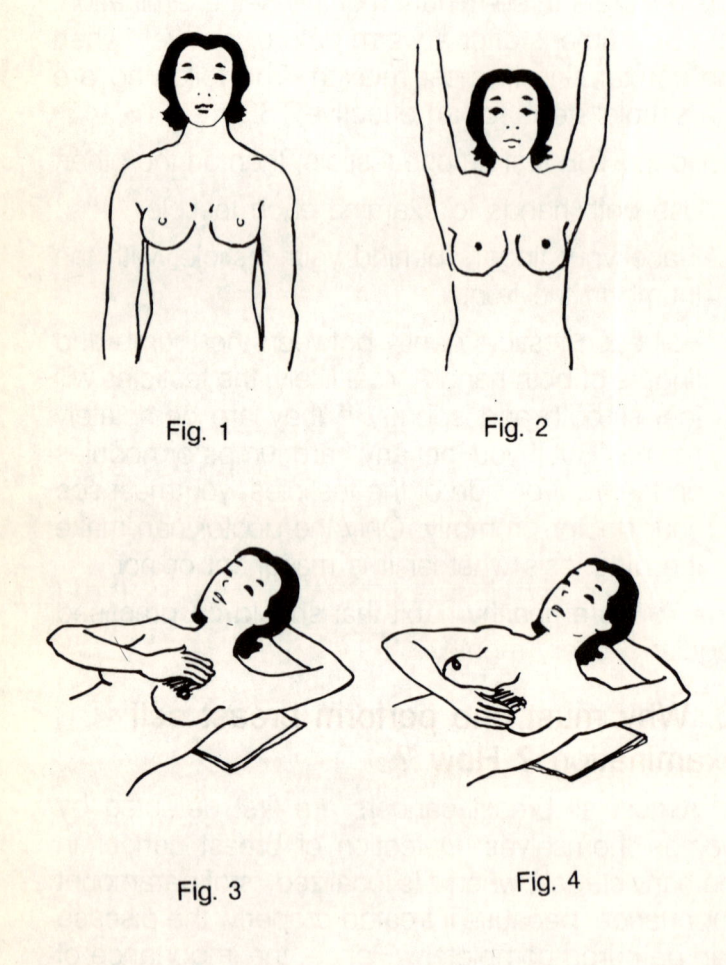

Fig. 2

Fig. 3

Fig. 4

Fig. 5

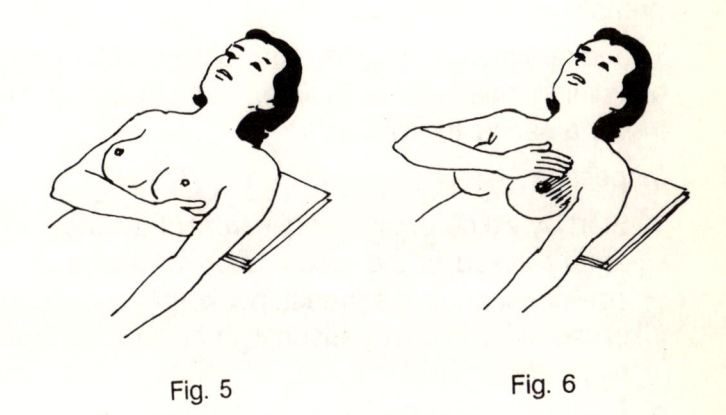

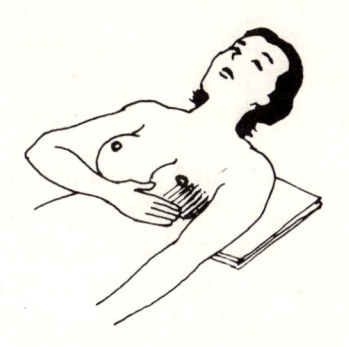

Fig. 6

Fig. 7

same time every month, just after the monthly period, when the breast is least likely to be nodular. One must look for any changes since the last time the breasts were examined.

The examination may be performed as follows, examining one side at a time, first inspecting and then palpating the breast.

Inspection –

1. Start by sitting or standing in front of a mirror, with arms relaxed at the sides. Look for a change in size or shape of the breast, puckering or dimpling of the skin, and any discharge or change in the nipple (Fig. 1).
2. Next, look for exactly the same things, after raising both arms over the head.

   The inspection is now complete and one may proceed to palpation of the breast, looking for any lump or thickening (Fig. 2).

Palpation –

1. Lie down and put a pillow under the left shoulder, with the left hand under the head. Using the fingers of the right hand, held together and flat, press gently but firmly with small circular movements, to feel the upper inner quarter of the breast, starting at the breast bone and going outward till you reach the nipple line. Feel the region around the nipple (Fig. 3).
2. Similarly, examine the lower inner part of the breast. In this region, a ridge of firm tissue may be felt which is normal (Fig. 4).

3. Now, bringing the hand down to the side, still using the fingers, feel under the armpit (Fig. 5).
4. After this, examine the upper outer quarter of the breast from the nipple line to where your arm is resting, in a similar manner (Fig. 6).
5. Lastly, with the same gentle pressure examine the lower outer quarter of the breast, starting from the outer part and going to the nipple (Fig. 7).

Repeat the same on the other side completing the examination of the breasts.

Thus, one broadly looks for a lump, change in the size or shape, puckering, dimpling or any other skin lesion over the breast and any change or discharge from the nipple.

If any abnormality is detected do not be alarmed, as all lumps or other changes are not cancers. However, it is best to consult a doctor for a complete and proper evaluation of the condition. Remember, breast cancer is curable and an early diagnosis can make all the difference with respect to the prognosis of a given case. Self examination of the breasts for early detection of cancers must be developed as a health habit which should be continued life long.

Q. What literature do you advise your patients to read ?

A. A well-informed patient is a better patient from all points of view. I would like to suggest the following books:

1. Human Sexual Response by Masters and Johnson
2. Human Sexual Inadequacy by Masters and

Johnson

3. The Joy of Sex by Alex Comfort
4. Illustrated Manual of Sex Therapy by H.S. Kaplan

Q. What advise would you give for a better sex life ?

A. Sexual literacy is the primary requirement for a good sex life. Do not be under pressure to perform or respond. Try to get familiar with your own and your partner's anatomy. Communicate mutual likes and dislikes. Adequate communication is vital for a healthy and mutually satisfying sex life. Avoid being monotonous. Be innovative and try different positions. Devote adequate time for foreplay and afterplay. Remember sensual is sexual.

Avoid stress, smoking and alcohol. Proper weight, balanced diet, regular exercises and yoga are essential for a better sex life. What is good for the whole body is good for sex.

15

MISCELLANEA

Q. How do quacks operate ?

A. Quacks are unqualified, so-called professionals who offer empirical, standard, constant therapy for all possible sexual disorders. They thrive on age old prevalent myths and misconceptions. I quote from what my patients have reported. After the patient has related his problem, the so-called sexologist immediately remarks: "Oh! it appears that you have masturbated a lot in the past, and that has led to a tremendous weakness in your genitals". They scare them further by saying that if they do not take their sex tonic courses, they would be incompetent for marriage. Some might 'conclude', by superficial examination, that they have lost a lot of 'highly precious' semen and would need to take long courses of sex tonics and rejuvenators to regain their lost vitality! Most quacks are blissfully unaware of the existence of female sexual dysfunctions and always put the onus on the male. Others arbitrarily brand female patients as frigid.

Some use a sort of electric instrument. They run it over all parts of the body; the instrument lights up indicating that there is enough flow of blood. As soon as it comes to the genitals they switch off the light by some mechanism, thereby indicating that there is a defect in flow of blood and, to restore this, they would have to resort to a sex tonic or rejuventor. Some openly advertise and create fear in the minds of gullible people thereby enticing them to their clinics and exploiting them.

As long as there are misconceptions, quacks will continue to thrive! As long as there are quacks, misconceptions will continue to thrive! Sex education, is the only answer to this horrendous 'cause and effect' relationship.

Q. Why don't you follow Masters and Johnson's model ?

A. Masters and Johnson treat a couple for two weeks. A majority of the couples take a vacation for two weeks and go for the treatment keeping away from their families. Evaluation is done in the initial days of the two weeks' active treatment. I followed a similar procedure but there were a number of subjects who had evidence of an organic cause responsible for the sexual dysfunction. That apart, several patients had psychiatric disorders; their depressions were severe, paranoia were pervasive, marital hostilities malignant and defenses rigid. Sex therapy, as practised all over the world, is contraindicated in a majority of these cases. It is easy to argue that, as these cases were referred, they were already evaluated by the family physicians. Is it possible for a family physician to go into details of the marital history, psychological background, symptoms suggestive of psychiatric illnesses and a thorough physical examination in his busy schedule ? Not in India, at least. Organic problems responsible for sexual dysfunction are many. The incidence of organic problems in our country is higher because of the poor health of the population and lack of regular medical check-ups. For example, phimosis or tight foreskin is not a rare condition seen in practice which can lead to sexual difficulty and at times sexual dysfunctions.

Vacations are really precious and in two weeks' active treatment, the Masters and Johnson's model has the hazard of further disappointing the already disappointed couple if there is any evidence of organic or major psychiatric illness. And finally, Masters & Johnson mention that they treat a relationship and not an individual... Is it possible to transform a relationship in two weeks' time ?

Q. What are the inadequacies of the existing classifications ?

A. Contemporary sexual medical literature though exhaustive, has persistently failed to realize the larger perspective of the all important event of orgasm. There is no well defined concept of orgasm as a separate entity though it has been conclusively established that orgasm – (a subjective cognitive pleasurable event) and ejaculation/vaginal contractions (an objective pelvic physiological event) are psychophysiodynamically distinct and discrete events, which in their undisputed duality, occur in close mutual temporal proximity. This terminological equation of orgasm = ejaculation/vaginal contractions was initially put forward by Masters and Johnson, the pioneers of sexual medical science. The emphasis on ejaculation (probably reflecting our inherent survival instinct) has been accepted by all subsequent researchers and scientists in this field (reflecting our herd instinct). The denial of the pleasure aspect of sexuality suggests a myopic, anhedonic, orthodox attitude, reminiscent of the sex negative pseudoreligious authoritarianism prevailing during the prudish victorian era.

Existing classifications based on this fundamental postulate which is erroneous, lead to conceptual pandemonium. Confusing, paradoxical and often multiple terminologies exist for the same disorders, while at the same time clinically different disorders may be clubbed together under a single 'terminological straitjacket'. The first hurdle in the study of orgasm is our inability to demonstrate an objective parameter which is the sine qua non of orgasm. Therefore, adapting to the dictates of our inadequacy, in true Orwellian style, contemporary sexual medicine recognizes studies and continues to perpetuate a scientific travesty!

There is a very constricted representation of female sexuality in contemporary sexual medicine and female sexual disorders are only cursorily dealt with.

Thus, existing sexual medicine is essentially utilitarian (procreation) in its outlook whereas, ideally a more totalitarian (pleasure + procreation) perspective is required. When considering the relative importance of the subjective pleasure *vis-à-vis* the objective parameter, one must realize that ejaculation/vaginal contractions merely represents a singular phenomenon in a whole spectrum of events, the objective of which is the orgasm.

One can summarize the inadequacies of the existing classifications for males by saying that they revolve around a 'pseudoprinciple' (ejaculation = orgasm), stressing only the 'pseudoprincipal' (ejaculation) de-stressing the 'principal principle' of the 'pleasure principle' (orgasm). The 'de-stress' on female sexuality and female sexual disorders, is also distressing to note. Both orgasm and female sexuality, should be given the greater consideration, that they merit, and should not be compromised because of our lack of scientific and lingual expressivity.

Q. How do you evaluate a case of sexual dysfunction ?

A. I evaluate sexual dysfunctions by inquiring about the cardinal parameters of desire, erection/lubrication, intromission, orgasm and ejaculation in the history taking. This covers every possible facet of the problem and helps in quickly localizing the dysfunction to a particular parameter. This method that I have evolved on my own, is both rapid and accurate, and is very effective clinically, even while examining a large volume of patients, on an out patient basis, at a general hospital, in a limited time span.

Desire : Desire could decrease in situations like depression, schizophrenia, dislike of the partner's body odour, fatigue, illness or disturbed inter-personal relationship. Desire could increase in conditions like mania, schizophrenia and sometimes following epilepsy or head injury.

Erection : If a man has a good quality of erection in any one situation i.e. in the morning or during masturbation, but not at the time of coitus, then the problem is largely situational (psychological) and not constitutional (organic).

Lubrication : The common causes of inadequate lubrication (at the time of coitus) are lack of adequate foreplay and arousal, local infections or hormonal imbalance. The most common cause is functional and must be ruled out before considering other causes.

Intromission : If a man is unable to penetrate, then his knowledge about the sexual position and female sexual anatomy should be inquired into. If there is evidence of pain at the time of penetration, then one must look for either phimosis and/or obstructive vaginal pathology. Often, having failed once, the fear of another failure coupled with performance anxiety, paralyses the sexual response, causing the erection to subside before intromission. After penetration, if the penis loses its firmness then, once again, the fear of failure or a lax vagina leading to inadequate peno-vaginal contact could be the cause.

Orgasm : Whether one has ever experienced orgasm during waking hours, or has any difficulty or delay in reaching orgasm or is reaching orgasm early should be inquired into; and depending upon the answers a diagnosis can be arrived at: viz. Absent, Impaired, Delayed or Early Orgasmic Response.

Ejaculation : Following orgasm, the ejaculate usually comes out through the urethral meatus – antegrade ejaculation. At times, following orgasm there is no ejaculation of semen outside – a dry run; this is usually known as retrograde ejaculation. Inquiry about the flow of semen (squirting or oozing) and simultaneous experience of pleasure needs to be made to identify the etiology.

Q. What is your opinion about the popular Ayurvedic herbal sex tonics ?

A. The basic principles of the Ayurvedic medical science are compromised at every stage in the making and administration of these 'Ayurvedic Herbal

Sex Tonics' that are popularly in use today. This can be verified from most authentic ayurvedic texts, including Charak samhita by Charak, Shushrut samhita by Shushrut and Ashtangrhaday by Vaghbhatt, among many others. I will try to enumerate and explain the various reasons why.

Principle

Today, ayurvedic herbal medicines are empirically prescribed for their supposed 'tonic' effect. Often, any one particular drug, is used in the treatment of all sexual dysfunctions. It is important to realize that different sexual dysfunctions cannot possibly have a singular etiology. Hence, the empirical therapeutic use of a single particular preparation for disorders of various etiologies cannot be justified. Ayurvedic texts mention that, without knowing the physiology (prakruti) or pathology (vikruti) of an individual (which is not possible without a detailed and devoted study of Ayurveda), it is dangerous and sometimes lethal to empirically prescribe any drug. These texts, specifically advise the use of different preparations for different disorders emphasizing that individualization and rationalization are a must for therapy to be successful and free of side effects.

Growth

Ayurvedic texts mention that, for herbs to be therapeutically efficacious they have to be grown on a particular type of land, and in a natural way with natural manures only. Today, the herbs are grown on any available land, alongwith the use of artificial fertilizer to enrich the soil and increase the yield of crop. This practice is at odds with the ayurvedic principles which categorically prohibit the use of any artificial means. Hence, it decreases drug efficacy and may even prove to be harmful.

Collection

Ayurvedic texts specify that different drugs have to be collected during different phases in the lunar cycle, which I doubt is being practised today.

Storage

Ayurveda stresses that after preparation, different medicines should be stored in different containers (usually glass or earthenware, containers unless specified otherwise) to preserve their efficacy, whereas today the majority of herbal 'tonics' available are stored either in gelatin capsules of animal origin, or aluminium foil or plastic containers. This casts serious doubts on their alleged efficacy as it is impossible to determine the drug interaction and hence drug potency due to the compromise of ayurvedic concepts and principles.

Duration of efficacy

Ayurvedic herbal medicines have specific expiry dates (usually 3 to 6 months) after which they lose their potency and become useless. Moreover, this date is to be considered with respect to the date when the herb was plucked and not the date of manufacture by the pharmaceutical company. It is surprising that there is no mention of an expiry date on the cover of most of the popular ayurvedic sex tonics. Further, I seriously doubt that the date of plucking of the herb is ever considered by those who do mention a date of expiry, of the herbal medicine.

Administration

Ayurvedic experts state that 'a dye cannot be properly applied over a dirty cloth and so is the case for medicines to be effective!' Thus, ayurveda requires the purification of body system (panchakarma) for the desired tonic effect (Vajeekaran). However, in direct contravention to this, today, no such purification of the body system is advocated, prior to the use of these tonics, not even a purge.

Sometimes, patients are advised to use ghee and honey, in equal proportions alongwith their medicines. 'Shushrut' has clearly stated that the use of ghee and honey in equal proportions is poisonous!

Ayurvedically speaking, the incongruity between the 'pre-scribed' ayurvedic principles and concepts and the empirical (ab)use of ayurvedic sex tonics, prescribed today, is too vast for them to be of any therapeutic value.

Q. What are the psychological sequelae of a rape case ?

A. The psychological trauma experienced in a rape case often exceeds the physical trauma. The affected individual loses her sense of self confidence and self esteem and becomes increasingly aware of her vulnerability. She develops negative attitudes towards sex. This will affect her response and performance in subsequent sexual encounters. Some victims avoid sexual intimacy and even if they do indulge, often recreate and relive the traumatic experience and are unable to continue the encounter. Sometimes orthodox society also considers the victim as promiscuous, who has probably invited the tragedy upon herself. She also becomes the object of the unsolicited attention of males looking for a casual temporary relationship. This could result in a further loss of self esteem and is psychologically detrimental.

♀♂

AFTERFACE

True to our legacy of a traditional social honesty from an ancient cultural past, I have approached the subject with a frankness, honesty and objectivity, which I believe are absolutely necessary because of the very nature of the subject itself.

Index

AFTERPLAY 63

AIDS 127

— AIDS 127
— Anal sex 128
— Prevention 129
— Safe practices 130

ALCOHOL 120

— Effect on sexual function 122
— Impotence 24
— Pregnancy 47

ALTERNATIVE ORIENTATIONS 75

— Alternative Orientations 75
— Bisexuality 76
— Lesbianism 76
— Homosexuality 75
— Paraphilias – See Paraphilias 77
— Transsexualism 79

APHRODISIACS 119

— Action 120
— Alcohol 120, 122
— Aphrodisiac 119
— Cocaine 123
— Ginseng 122
— Marijuana 122
— Paan 125
— Papaverine 125
— Testosterone 123, 124

AYURVEDIC HERBAL SEX TONICS 149

BISEXUALITY – See Alternative Orientations 75

BREAST 42

— Disparity 43
— Enlargement 43
— Exercises 43
— Hair 44
— Implants 44
— Sagging 43
— Self examination 137
— Size 43
— Stimulation 42
— Stretch marks 47

BULBOURETHRAL GLANDS

— See Cowper's Glands 28

CELIBACY 16

CIRCUMCISION 38

— Female 49

— Newborn male 38
— Orgasmic control 39

CLITORIS 44

— Adhesions 45
— Climax 45
— Stimulation 45

CONTRACEPTION 105

— Coitus interruptus 107
— Condom 107
— Different methods 106
— IUCD 108
— Oral pills 109
  — Contraindications 110
  — Mechanism 110
  — Misconceptions 109
— Post coital 111
— Suppositories 108
— Tubectomy 117
  — Desire 117
  — Hormonal level 117
  — Reversal 117
— Vasectomy 111
  — Acceptance 116
  — Complications 113
  — Contraindications 113
  — Desire 115
  — Hormonal levels 114
  — Precautions 114
  — Residual sperms 114
  — Reversal 116

COWPER'S GLANDS 28

DESIRE 96

— After – tubectomy 117
        – vasectomy 115
— Decrease 96
— Excessive 96
— Menopause 82

DHAT SYNDROME 14

DOPPLER EXAMINATION 26

DYSPAREUNIA 68

ELECTROMYOGRAPHY (EMG) 26

EPISIOTOMY 48

ERECTION

— Elderly 81
— Local stimulation 61
— Painful 28
— Peyronie's disease 91
— Role of anxiety 24

EROTIC LITERATURE 67

EUNUCHS 79

EXTRAMARITAL AFFAIRS

— See Marriage 101

FAMILY PLANNING – See Contraception 105

FANTASY 67

FOREPLAY – See Interplay 63

FREQUENCY 65

G-SPOT 45

HOMOSEXUALITY — See Alternative Orientations 75

ILL HEALTH 87

— AIDS – see AIDS 127
— Arthritis 92
— Back pain 93
— Blood pressure 89
  — Medication 90
— Bronchial asthma 90
— Diabetes 87
— Heart disease 88
  — Precautions 88, 89

— Hysterectomy   95
— Jaundice   92
— Kidney disease   91
— Mastectomy   94
— Obesity   95
— Peyronies disease   91
— Prostate operation   94
— Smoking   95

IMPOTENCE   24

— Causes   25
— Investigations   26
— Semen analysis   25
— Use of penile implants   27
— Xrays, leading to   96

INTERPLAY   63

— Afterplay   63
— Foreplay   63
— Intercourse   64
  — Anal sex   73
  — Duration   64
  — Frequency   65
  — Oral sex   73
  — Pain (Dyspareunia)   68
  — Positions   44, 70, 71, 72
  — Vaginismus   68

LESBIANISM   76

— See Alternative Orientations   75

LITERATURE ON SEX   141

MARRIAGE   99

— Disturbed marital harmony   102
— Extramarital affair   101
— Marriage   99
— Sex   99, 100
— Stress   100

MASTERS AND JOHNSON'S MODEL   144

MASTURBATION   10

— After marriage   102
— Curvature of penis   13
— Excess   11
— Female   10
— Male   10
— Parents' reaction   12
— Treatment   11

MENOPAUSE   82

— Desire   82
— Use of estrogens   85

MENSTRUATION   135

— Sex   135
— Use of condom   135

NOCTURNAL PENILE TUMESCENCE (NPT)   126

OBESITY   95

ORGASM   53

— Clitoral stimulation   60
— Circumcision   49
— Diaphragm   60
— Different names   58
— Erogenous zones   60
— Genital stimulation   61
— Identification   59
— Mechanism   55
— Multiorgasm
  – Female   62
  – Male   62
— Orgasmic dysfunctions   54
— Physical signs   59
— Simultaneous   20
— Why   54

ORGASMIC CONTROL 32

PAPAVERINE 125

— Injection 125
— Side effect 125

PARAPHILIAS 77

— Exhibitionism 78
— Fetishism 77
— Frottage 78
— Gerontophilia 79
— Masochism 78
— Necrophilia 79
— Pedophilia 77
— Sadism 78
— Transvestism 77
— Voyeurism 78
— Zoophilia 77

PENILE BLOOD PRESSURE 26

PENILE IMPLANT 27

PENIS

— Circumcision 38, 39
— Curvature 13, 20
— Length 17
— Masturbation 13
— Pain on erection 28
— Phimosis 28, 30
— Width 19

PHIMOSIS 28

PREGNANCY 46

— Abortion 46
— Alcohol 47
— Episiotomy 48
— Pleasure 48
— Positions 46
— Precautions 46
— Sex – during 46
    – after 47
— Smoking 47
— Stretch marks 47
— Vaginal laxity 48, 49
— Virgin 46

PREMATURE EJACULATION 30

PROSTATE 85

— Benign hyperplasia 85
— Operation 94

QUACKS 143

RAPE 153

SEMEN 13

— Colour 14
— Conservation 13
— Consistency 13
— Analysis in impotence 25
— Excessive dissipation 13
— In urine 14
— Quantity 14
— Seeping from vagina 68

SEX

— Abstinence 16
— Anal 73
— Different positions 70
— Effects of work situations
    — adverse 104
    — favourable 103
— Excess Desire 96
— Oral 73
— Without coitus 65

SEX EDUCATION 1

— Abuse, sexual 6
— How 3
— Parents' role 3,4,5,12
— When 2
— Why 2

— Use of media   7

SEX TONICS

— See Aphrodisiacs   119

SEXUAL MYTHS   9

— Celibacy   16
— Dhat syndrome   14
— Masturbation   10
— Penis   17
— Sleep emissions   16
— Value of semen   13
— Virginity   20

SLEEP EMISSIONS   16

— Weakness   16

SQUEEZE TECHNIQUE   37

TESTIS   23, 24

— Self examination   136
— Single   23

TESTOSTERONE   123

— In elderly   124

— In sexual dysfunctions   123
— What is   123

TOWARDS HEALTHY SEXUALITY   133

— Sexual hygiene   133
— Tampoon   134
— To clean private parts   133
— Vaginal douche/deodorant   134

VAGINA

— Laxity   48, 49
— Lubrication – excessive   46

VAGINAL DOUCHE   134

VAGINISMUS   68

— What is   68
— Treatment   68

VIBRATORS   135, 136

VIRGINITY   41, 20

VIRILITY   14

Dear Reader,

Your comments will be gratefully acknowledged. If you have any further questions or difficulties or if you feel any more questions are inadvertently omitted which should have been included in this book, kindly fill in the proforma given below and mail to:

Prof. Prakash Kothari
203 A Sukh Sagar
N.S. Patkar Marg
Bombay 400 007
India

Name and address:
(Optional)

Comments/Questions: